STATISTICAL METHODS IN PSYCHIATRY RESEARCH AND SPSS

STATISTICAL METHODS IN PSYCHIATRY RESEARCH AND SPSS

M. Venkataswamy Reddy, PhD

Apple Academic Press

TORONTO   NEW JERSEY

Apple Academic Press Inc. | Apple Academic Press Inc.
3333 Mistwell Crescent | 9 Spinnaker Way
Oakville, ON L6L 0A2 | Waretown, NJ 08758
Canada | USA

©2015 by Apple Academic Press, Inc.

First issued in paperback 2021

Exclusive worldwide distribution by CRC Press, a member of Taylor & Francis Group
No claim to original U.S. Government works

ISBN 13: 978-1-77463-351-9 (pbk)
ISBN 13: 978-1-77188-035-0 (hbk)

Library of Congress Control Number: 2014946042

Library and Archives Canada Cataloguing in Publication

Reddy, M. Venkataswamy, author
Statistical methods in psychiatry research and SPSS/M. Venkataswamy Reddy, PhD.

Includes bibliographical references and index.
ISBN 978-1-77188-035-0 (bound)
1. Psychiatry--Research--Statistical methods. 2. SPSS (Computer file). I. Title.

RC337.R38 2014   616.89'00727   C2014-905178-6

Apple Academic Press also publishes its books in a variety of electronic formats. Some content that appears in print may not be available in electronic format. For information about Apple Academic Press products, visit our website at **www.appleacademicpress.com** and the CRC Press website at **www.crcpress.com**

ABOUT THE AUTHOR

M. Venkataswamy Reddy, PhD

M. Venkataswamy Reddy is a permanent faculty member at the National Institute of Mental Health and Neuro Sciences (NIMHANS), Bangalore, India, and has over 30 years of teaching experience. He has published more than 20 scientific papers. His popular textbook, titled *Statistics for Mental Health Care Research*, is widely referred to by students and academicians alike. His main contributions include the development of suitable models for mental health delivery systems in India, meta-analysis for psychiatry research and STATA, and cluster analysis for psychiatry research and SPSS. He received an MSc in statistics from the Department of Statistics at Bangalore University; a DBS (PG diploma in Biostatistics) from ICMR's Institute for Research in Medical Statistics, New Delhi; and a PhD in Biostatistics (topic: cluster formation in psychiatry with special reference to child psychiatry) from Bangalore University.

CONTENTS

LIST OF ABBREVIATIONS

AGR	annual growth rate
ANCOVA	analysis of covariance
ANOVA	analysis of variance
CDR	crude death rate
CI	confidence interval
CRD	completely randomized design
CV	coefficient of variation
DOS	duration of stay
DSD	dissociative disorder
DV	dependent variable
ECT	electroconvulsive therapy
FN	false negative
IPSS	Indian Psychiatric Survey Schedule
IQ	intelligent quotient
MANOVA	multivariate analysis of variance
NIMHANS	The National Institute of Mental Health and Neurosciences
OCD	obsessive and compulsive disorder
OR	odds ratio
OTD	obsessive thought disorder
PCI	per capita income
RBD	randomized block design
RPES	rapid psychiatric examination schedule
RR	risk ratio
SE	standard error
SES	socio-economic status
SOM	somatoform
SPSS	statistical package for social sciences
TP	true positive

PREFACE

This book is best suited for professionals, teachers, and post-graduate students in the fields of psychiatry and allied mental health such as psychiatric social work, psychiatric nursing, psychiatric epidemiology, psychiatric statistics, mental health education, and clinical psychology. Keeping a watchful eye on the perfection of knowledge of these methods, this book has been prepared with a view to fill gaps in their applications and to introduce suitable data analysis software. The main objectives of writing this book include classification of fundamental statistical methods in psychiatry research, introduction to multivariate data analysis, and data analysis software presented in a precise and simple manner.

Hierarchical classification of the contents: The sequence of the 22 chapters, the sections within the chapters, the subsections within the sections, and the points listed under these subsections have been so arranged to help the professionals in classification of their knowledge in statistical methods (see Appendix II) and fill the gaps. The reader can make a glossary by referring to the meanings and definitions of the various terms given in the appendix to the main text of the book. This appendix can also provide an index.

Precise: My intension is to provide an overview of statistical methods, but the works that I have found most useful are included in the bibliography. This feature of the book helps the reader, who merely requires having his memory refreshed, in preparing a summary of statistical formula from the text of the book.

Simplicity: The fundamental statistical methods are demonstrated by means of arithmetical examples that may be reworked with pencil and paper in a matter of minutes. Most of these examples use artificial data: real data are usually more difficult to work with and can easily obscure the point being made. Care has been taken to avoid using terminology that is likely to cause difficulty to the reader.

Data analysis software: The results of the rework by the reader have to be checked by using SPSS; and in this way, the psychiatrist friendly data analysis software (SPSS) is introduced.

ACKNOWLEDGMENT

I am grateful to Dr. P. Satishchandra, Director/Vice Chancellor, National Institute of Mental Health and Neurosciences (NIMHANS), Bangalore, India, for the support and encouragement during the preparation of this manuscript. I thank Dr. Mallikarjun B. Hanji and Dr. K. P. Suresh for rendering enormous help by going through the manuscript and assisting in the preparation of the solutions of the exercises. I thank Shri Ashish Kumar of Apple Academic Press for his full cooperation in bringing out the book in its present nice form.

This book is the first of its kind. Critical examination and suggestions to improve the book from any corner will be appreciated.

M. Venkataswamy Reddy

CHAPTER 1

PSYCHIATRIC RESEARCH

CONTENTS

1.1   RESEARCH QUESTIONS IN PSYCHIATRY

1.1.1   RECOGNITION

In recognizing cases (screening), the research questions may arise in the following areas:
1. Documentation of natural history of various psychiatric disorders/ diseases
2. Definitions of abnormal conditions

1.1.2   DIAGNOSIS

In diagnosing the recognized patients, the research questions may arise in the following areas:
1. Documentation of disease processing and mechanism
2. Disease description
3. Making diagnosis
4. Predicting the prognosis of the diagnosed patients

1.1.3   TREATMENT

In treating the diagnosed patients, the research questions may arise in the following areas:
1. Documentation of medical/therapeutic history of various psychiatric diseases
2. Planning of clinical trials; evaluation of different levels of the treatment; and providing standard measures of accuracy of various clinical procedures
3. Promotion of adequate clinical facilities
4. Determining the outcome of the treated cases

1.1.4   PREVENTION

In preventing diseases/disorders, the research questions may arise in the following areas:

1. Assessing of the state of mental health in the community and indication of the basic factors underlying this state of mental health in the community
2. Finding out the risk/causal factors associated with various psychiatric diseases
3. Planning and monitoring of mental health programs for specific population groups and evaluation of the total program of action
4. Promotion of mental health legislation

1.2   RESEARCH APPROACHES

1.2.1   SCIENTIFIC APPROACH

Scientific approach is the application of logic and objectivity in order to understand the phenomenon. When two mental health workers adapt this approach, both will arrive at the same conclusion with the same data in recognizing cases, making diagnosis of the patient, deciding on the course and method of treatment, predicting the outcome of the treatment, and in determining the cause of a mental disorder to prevent them. This is because of the standard features and steps involved in the scientific method.

1.2.1.1   FEATURES

The scientific method has several specific features such as the circularity aspect of facts and theory, humility, free inquiry, free from human bias, controlled observation, comparability, repeatability, ruling out metaphysical explanations, and the use of both inductive and deductive reasoning.

1.2.1.2   STEPS

The following five steps are involved in the scientific method: formulation of problem, formulation of hypotheses, modification of the problem/hypotheses, testing (verification or experimentation), and generalization.

1.2.1.3   SCIENCE AND PSYCHIATRY

In order to be called as a scientific discipline, the field of psychiatry has undergone the rigors of various non-scientific approaches to acquire knowledge such as the method of tenacity (blind belief), the method of authority (established belief), and the method of intuition (a priori method). Thus, psychiatry is the oldest art and newest science.

1.2.2   MILL'S CANONS

Statistics is used to determine causal factors of phenomena in experimental inquiries. John Stuart Mill presented logical devices as short rules under the title "methods of experimental inquiry." These rules indicate five canons.

1.2.2.1   METHOD OF DIFFERENCE

This consists in making use of two groups of subjects equal in all respects and do something to one of the groups (experimental group) and not doing anything to the other group (control group). If a change takes place in some dependent variable in the experimental group, but it does not take place in the control group, then the change in the dependent variable is attributed to the manipulation in the experimental group.

Example: Let us suppose that 60 schizophrenic patients are randomly divided into two groups of 30 patients in each group. One group is given educational input along with the treatment, and the other group is given the treatment without additional educational input. The educational input group has demonstrated better understanding of the illness which led to better follow-ups and management.

1.2.2.2   METHOD OF AGREEMENT

Whenever the researcher observes the occurance of phenomenon, he must notice presence of specific independent and dependent variables. This consists in observing the occurrence of the phenomenon in each time where a specific independent variable presents, a specific dependent variable occurs. The researcher continues to observe the occurrence of the phenomenon with different combinations of his independent variable until he ascertains that there is only one specific independent variable that always presents whenever a specific dependent variable occurred. Then, he would infer that the independent variable that was common to the occurrence is related to the occurrence of the dependent variable.

Example: The case history records of 28 conduct disorder children revealed that all of them had either inadequate parental control or family over involvement. By applying the method of agreement, it is possible to state a relationship between the occurrence of conduct disorder and the presence of inadequate parental control or family over involved.

1.2.2.3   JOINT METHOD OF DIFFERENCE AND AGREEMENT

This method consists in testing to see that if in two or more instances, the phenomenon has only one factor in common and then test to see that if in two or more instances where that common factor is absent, the phenomenon does not occur. The researcher concludes that the common factor is related to the occurrence of the phenomenon.

*Example:*The case history records of 200 child guidance clinic children revealed that all the 23 children with hyperkinetic disorder had abnormal attention and concentration, and only two of the remaining children had this abnormality. Hence, it can be said that certain relationship may exist between the occurrence of hyperkinetic disorders and the presence of abnormal attention/concentration in children.

1.2.2.4   METHOD OF CONCOMITANT VARIATION

This method consists in recording the variation of both the independent variable and the dependent variable; and if the dependent variable varies in any manner whenever the independent variable varies in some particular manner, the experimenter concludes that the two variables are related.

*Example:*The findings of mental morbidity studies carried out in India revealed several relationships between the prevalence of mental/behavioral disorders and several biosocial variables. The findings further indicate that the risk of mental and behavioral disorders of a person decreases with increased socio-economic status, increases gradually up to 40 years of age and decreases thereafter, and increases with both the size of his family,urbanization of his locality, etc.

1.2.2.5   METHOD OF RESIDUES

This method consists in attempting to determine, through experimentation and deduction, the phenomena that are due to the effect of the presence of specific and identifiable independent variables. The researcher continues to ascertain such information until the relationship between one dependent variable and one independent variable is unknown in the situation. Then, the investigator infers that this remaining independent variable is related to the remaining dependent variable.

Example: A series of five drugs are administered to a group of patients and the responses are noted down. Then, each drug is withdrawn every time from least important to most important in order to find out at which withdrawal of the drug the patients stop improving or regressing.

1.2.3   QUALITATIVE RESEARCH

Qualitative research involves collecting qualitative data by way of in-depth interviews, open-ended questions, observations, and field notes. The researcher is the primary source of data collection, and the data could be collected in the form of words, images, and pattern. Data analysis involves searching for pattern, themes, and holistic features. Results of such research are context specific, and reporting takes the form of a narrative with contextual descriptions and direct quotation from researchers.

1.2.4   QUANTITATIVE RESEARCH

Quantitative research involves collecting quantitative data based on precise measurements using structured, reliable, and validated data collection instruments or through archival data sources. The nature of the data is in the form of variables. Based on the purpose of the study, the studies of quantitative research can be broadly classified as observational studies and experimental studies.

1.3 PROTOCOL WRITING FOR QUANTITATIVE STUDIES

1.3.1 THE RESEARCH QUESTION

1.3.1.1 REVIEW OF LITERATURE

A research question/problem arises in two occasions:first, to develop a theory to explain an event that occurred, and none of the existing theories explained it so for and second, to modify the existing theory so as to suit the new event.In order to identify the problem, the scientist must have good acquaintance with the area in which he has to identify the problem. Thus, he has to review the relevant literature (standard authors' work).

1.3.1.2 NEED FOR THE STUDY

The need for the study is an important consideration as it specifies the priority to be given and the budget that is required for the study.

1.3.1.3 AIMS AND OBJECTIVES

The aim of the study is to find out the truth that is hidden and that has not been discovered so far. The objectives of the study are to discover answers to questions using scientific procedures. According to the nature of the objectives, the studies may be classified as exploratory to gain familiarity with a phenomenon, descriptive to portray accurately the characteristics of a particular group, hypothesis testing to test a hypothesis of a causal relationship between variables, or diagnostic to determine the frequency with which something is associated with something else.

1.3.2 TYPE OF STUDY

The protocol writer has to specify the type of study, whether it is observational (case-series, cross-sectional, or longitudinal) or experimental (informal or formal).

1.3.3   PLAN OF STUDY

1.3.3.1   POPULATION

The term "population" has wider meaning in any research activity. It is the aggregate of units of observation about which certain information is required. When the investigation is carried out for all the units in the population, it is called census enumeration. The statistical constants based on population values are known as parameters. In psychiatric research, we are mainly concerned with populations such as the following:

1. General population of a defined community
2. Psychiatric patients at a particular point of time in the community
3. New psychiatric patients during a particular time period in the community
4. Out-patient registrations in a mental health delivery system during a time period (say 1 year)
5. Admitted patients in a mental health institution/general hospital psychiatric unit during a time period (say 1year)
6. All in-patients at a particular point of time in a mental health institute/general hospital psychiatric unit
7. Discharged patients during a particular time period.

1.3.3.2   VARIABLES

The characteristics on which the observations are made are known as variables such as age, sex, diagnosis, etc.

1.3.3.3   STANDARDISATION

All the terms/categories used in the study have to be clearly defined and standardized. For example, an urban locality may be defined as one with closed drainage facility, semi-urban as one with open drainage facility, and rural as one with no drainage facility. In mental health information system, a death in a hospital can be conveniently defined as a specific category of discharge.

1.3.3.4   EXPERIMENTAL (IF ANY)

The experimental setup (if any) is where a variable may be changed so that changes in the final output may be compared with the control setup. The control setup will be the basis of all measurements and a means of comparison.

1.3.3.5   RECORD FORM

In both observational studies and experimental studies, the investigator collects data by using a *proforma* that may be a questionnaire, schedule, or record form. In questionnaire approach, the respondents fill the *proforma* and return them or send them by post. In the schedule approach, the investigator asks specific questions and fills the *proforma*. The record forms are used to extract secondary data. Before the finalization of *proforma*, it is advantageous to carry out a pilot study on a small number of units. The results of the pilot study may be used to determine the sample size required for major studies.

1.3.3.6   RESPONSE ERROR

Response errors are the wrong or biased answers. The quality of the data collected may be assessed by cross checking. In experimental studies, the response errors are referred to as experimental errors.

1.3.3.7   NON-RESPONSE ERROR

Non-response errors mean failure to measure some of the units in the selected sample. Such errors may be minimized through adequate planning, training, monitoring, and supervision.

1.3.4   PLAN OF ANALYSIS

1.3.4.1   STATISTICAL METHODS

Statistical methods are the tools of science to deal with mass data. These are the mathematical devices of use in measuring variables/traits; discovering certain differences, relationships, probable predictions/trends, occurrence of events by time, and decomposition of seasonal variation; discovering distinct groups; identification of individuals; reduction of data, and synthesizing the results of similar studies. Based on probability scale, they help the researchers to decide whether these differences, relationships, trends, etc., are large enough to be considered as significant (real) or due to chance factor.

1.3.4.2   DATABASE AND DATA ANALYSIS SOFTWARE

A store of information often held on a computer as a database is stored as a number of records or files, each of which usually contains entries under a number of headings or fields. For example, a psychiatrist keeps a database under the following headings: name of the patient, age, sex, dateof visit, symptoms, diagnosis, treatment, etc. The ability of a computer to cross-reference within a database makes it a particularly efficient form for storing and handling data. It could, for example, be made to search the database for all patients suffering from schizophrenia.

The ready-made set of instructions called package have been developed, which can be used to carry out statistical analysis of the data. The statistical package for social sciences SPSS (Chapters 21 and 22) are the commonly used data analysis software in psychiatric research and allied fields.

1.3.5   REPORTING THE RESULTS

Before reporting the results, the study has to be evaluated and checked to see whether the results are correctly interpreted. The reporting of the results of scientific studies is different from those of the technical reports. The report must be reasonably brief, with tables and graphs when necessary, and reading the report should be a stimulating and satisfying experience.

1.4   VARIABLES IN PSYCHIATRY

1.4.1   NATURE OF VARIABLES IN PSYCHIATRY

1.   Demographic variables : age, sex, marital status, etc.
2.   Socio-cultural variables : religion/caste, region, domicile, etc.
3.   Socio-economic variables : education, occupation, income, etc.
4.   Family variables : family type, family structure, family size, etc.
5.   Signs and symptoms : hallucinations, delusions, etc.
6.   Diagnostic variables : schizophrenia, mania, etc.
7.   Treatment variables : psychotropic drugs, ECT, psychotherapy, etc.
8.   Hospitalization variables : hospitalization, duration of stay, etc.
9.   Outcome variables : type of discharge, result of treatment, etc.

1.4.2   QUALITATIVE AND QUANTITATIVE VARIABLES

A qualitative variable (sex, religion, diagnosis, etc.) is one in which the variables differ in kind rather than in magnitude. A qualitative variable may be dichotomous such as sex (male and female) or polychotomous such as religion (Hindu, Muslim, Christian, etc.). The categories (domain) of some of the important variables are sex (male, female, etc.), marital status (unmarried, married, widow/er, divorced, separated, remarried, etc.), religion (Hindu, Muslim, Christian, etc.), domicile (rural, semi-urban, urban), family type (nuclear, joint, extended, living together), and diagnosis (ICD-11).A quantitative variable (age, income, etc.) is one in which the variates differ in magnitude.

1.4.3   LEVELS OF MEASUREMENT OF VARIABLES

Qualitative (categorical) variables can be classified as nominal and ordinal variables according to the level of measurement. The quantitative variables (discrete or continuous) can be classified as interval-scale variables and ratio-scale variables.

1.4.3.1   NOMINAL LEVEL

Measurement in which a name is assigned to each observation belongs to the nominal scale of measurement. The variables such as sex, religion, diagnosis, etc., are measured in nominal scale of measurement.

1.4.3.2   ORDINAL LEVEL

The ordinal scale differs from the nominal scale in that it ranks the different categories specified in the scale in terms of a graded order. Variables such as severity of mental retardation (borderline, mild, moderate, severe, profound), and socio-economic status (low, middle, high) are measured in ordinal level/scale. Ranked variable is a special kind of ordinal variable in which the individual observations can be put in order from smallest to largest, even though the exact values are known.

1.4.3.3   INTERVAL LEVEL

The interval scale has all the characteristics of an ordinal scale.In addition, the distances between the successive scale points are of equal size. Variables such as intelligent quotient (IQ), achievement test scores, etc., are measured in interval scale of measurement. Here, zero point and the unit of measurement are arbitrary.

1.4.3.4   RATIO LEVEL

A ratio scale has all the characteristics of an interval scale; and in addition, it has an absolute zero point. Variables such as height, weight, etc., are measured in ratio scale. The scores obtained on psychosocial variables may be treated as if they are measured in ratio scale on the assumption that no serious errors will be incurred.

1.4.4   FURTHER TYPES OF VARIABLES

1.4.4.1   INDEPENDENT AND DEPENDENT VARIABLES

In psychiatric research, an independent variable is the factor that is chosen or manipulated by the experimenter in order to discover the effect on the dependent variable. A dependent variable is the factor that is observed or measured by the investigator-the outcome of the study.

1.4.4.2   COVARIATES

Covariates are interval-level independent variable. A covariate is a variable that is possibly predictive of the outcome under study. A covariate may be of direct interact or it may be a confounding one.

1.4.4.3   CONCOMITANT VARIABLES

A variable that is observed in a statistical experiment but that is not specially measured is called a concomitant variable. It is sometimes necessary to correct for concomitant variable in order to prevent distortion of the results of experiment or survey.

1.4.4.4   FACTORS/DIMENSIONS

Factors are nominal-level or ordinal-level independent variables.

1.4.5   DISCRETE AND CONTINUOUS DATA

Discrete data can only have specified values. The discrete data may be nominal data (male, female data), ordinal data (mild, moderate, severe data), ranking data, or whole number data. Continuous data are often referred to as measurement data. Continuous data can have any numerical value such as the height of a person.

1.5   STATISTICAL METHODS IN PSYCHIATRIC RESEARCH

The statistical methods selected for a particular study depend on the objectives of the study and the type of data collected for the purpose. These statistical methods can be broadly classified according to the number of variables that are simultaneously available for analysis (univariate statistical methods, bivariate statistical methods, and multivariate statistical methods).

1.5.1   ORGANIZATION AND COLLECTION OF DATA

1.5.1.1   OBSERVATIONAL STUDIES (CHAPTER 2)

Observational studies collect data from an existing situation.

1.5.1.2   EXPERIMENTAL STUDIES (CHAPTER 3)

Experimental studies are ones in which the investigator deliberately sets one or more factors at a specified level.

1.5.2   DESCRIPTIVE STATISTICS

1.5.2.1   ONE-VARIABLE DESCRIPTIVE STATISTICS (CHAPTER 4)

These methods portray accurately the characteristics such as the type of frequency distribution of observed values and summarization figures of the characteristics of the univariate data. Thus, it helps in gaining familiarity with the situations and phenomena.

1.5.2.2   MENTAL HEALTH STATISTICS (CHAPTER 5)

These are the descriptive statistics in the field of psychiatric service and research.

1.5.3 BASIS OF STATISTICAL INFERENCE

1.5.3.1 PROBABILITY AND PROBABILITY DISTRIBUTIONS (CHAPTER 6)

The probability scale is the basis of statistical inference. It includes both the estimation of parameters and test of significance of hypotheses. The descriptive statistics forms the material for statistical inference.

1.5.3.2 SAMPLING THEORY AND METHODS (CHAPTER 7)

These are the important steps in any research project as it is rarely practical, efficient, or ethical to study the whole population. The aim of random sampling approaches is to draw a representative sample from the population, so that the results of studying the sample can then be generalized back to the population. The selection of an appropriate method depends on the aim and objectives of the study and on the nature of the population to be studied.

1.5.3.3 BASIC ELEMENTS OF STATISTICAL INFERENCE (CHAPTER 8)

These elements include the estimation of parameters (criteria for selecting a suitable point estimators and interval estimators, and determining the sample size for drawing valid conclusions, etc.) and test of significance of hypotheses (formulation of hypotheses, level of significance, test statistics, etc.).

1.5.4 TESTS OF SIGNIFICANCE OF HYPOTHESES

1.5.4.1 PARAMETRIC TESTS OF SIGNIFICANCE (CHAPTER 9)

The parametric tests of significance are the test of hypothesis which assums that, the population is particular type of distribution (normal distribution) and test the value of one of the parameters. The parameter tested depends on the distribution. Examples : The normal test in the t-test for population mean, the use of correlation coefficient for the population correlation and the chi-square test for the population variance. These include the tests of significance of difference between means (arithmetic means) of groups on a variable facilitate whether the difference is significant (real) or due to merely a chance factor.

1.5.4.2   EXPERIMENTAL DATA ANALYSIS: ANOVA (CHAPTER 10)

These include the analysis of variance (ANOVA) tests of significance. These are the extension of parametric tests of significance for more than two groups.

1.5.4.3   NON-PARAMETRIC TESTS OF SIGNIFICANCE (CHAPTER 11)

These are the methods of inference in which there are no assumptions made about the nature, shape, or form of the population from which the data are obtained. They are preferred when the sample size is small and for qualitative variable data including ranking data or order data.

1.5.5   CORRELATIONAL VARIABLES DATA ANALYSIS

1.5.5.1   CORRELATIONAL ANALYSIS AND REGRESSION ANALYSIS (CHAPTER 12)

The correlation analysis measures the strength of correlation/association between variables and then test whether these correlations are significant or due to chance factor. On the contrary, the regression analysis fits functional relationship between dependent variable (e.g.the outcome of the treatment) and the independent variables (e.g. the type of treatment, etc.), and therefore it facilitates in predicting the value of the dependent variable based on the values of the independent variables.

1.5.5.2   RELIABILITY ANALYSIS AND VALIDITY ANALYSIS (CHAPTER 13)

Reliability is the consistency of a set of measurements or of a measuring instrument, which is often used to describe a test. Instrument validity is the degree to which an instrument measures what it is intended to measure.

1.5.5.3   SURVIVAL ANALYSIS AND TIME SERIES ANALYSIS (CHAPTER 14)

There are two aspects in time-related data analysis. Survival analysis deals with the estimation of probability (chance) of occurrence of events within a specified time period or estimation of time period for an event to occur. The time series analysis determines the influence of time components such as the trend, seasonal variation, and cyclical component on the occurrence of events, and thereby forecast the events.

1.5.6   MULTIVARIATE DATA ANALYSIS

1.5.6.1   MULTIVARIATE STATISTICAL METHODS (CHAPTER 15)

These methods simultaneously analyze more than two variables. These methods take into account the various correlations of the variables, and hence they give more realistic results.

1.5.6.2   CLUSTER ANALYSIS (CHAPTER 16)

These methods form groups of similar individuals (patients) and then establish the characteristics of the groups for the purpose of a classificatory system (ICD, DSM) or for any other research goals.

1.5.6.3   DISCRIMINANT ANALYSIS (CHAPTER 17)

These methods determine a set of characteristics that can significantly differentiate between the groups and in the process allocate individual objects (patients) into established classes (diagnostic categories) on the basis of specific criteria.

1.5.6.4   FACTOR ANALYSIS (CHAPTER 18)

Factor analysis involves grouping of similar variables (test items, signs, symptoms, etc.) to few factors or dimensions. The socio-economic status is based on education, occupation, and income. Thus, the factor analysis involves data reduction. The correlations between variables form the basic material for this purpose.

1.5.7   MULTI-STUDY DATA-POINTS ANALYSIS

1.5.7.1   META-ANALYSIS (CHAPTER 19)

The meta-analysis synthesizes (combine systematically) the results of similar but independent studies on a subject whenever several studies on a subject have conflicting conclusions.

KEYWORDS

- **Analysis of variance**
- **Dependent variable**
- **Hypothesis testing**
- **Independent variable**
- **Intelligent quotient**
- **Psychiatric disorders**
- **SPSS**

CHAPTER 2

OBSERVATIONAL STUDIES

CONTENTS

2.1   CASE-SERIES ANALYSIS

A case-series analysis report is a simple descriptive account of investigating characteristics observed in a group of registered patients.

2.1.1   OBSERVATIONAL UNITS

Observational units in a case-series analysis are the registered psychiatric patients in a mental health delivery system.

2.1.2   VARIABLES

The variables that are to be included in case-series analysis depend on the purpose of the study and the particular mental health delivery system. However, it is necessary to include important basic variables such as age, sex, and diagnosis.

2.1.3   RECORD FORM

In the record form, the rows represent the patients and the columns indicate the variables. The Appendix I illustrates a typical record form to collect data of registered psychiatric patients at NIMHANS hospital.

The case-series analysis is vital because of its descriptive role as precursors to other studies. The observations from such studies may be extremely useful to investigator in designing a study to evaluate cause or explanations of the observations. They should be viewed as hypotheses generating and not as causative. The appropriate statistical methods to analyze the data in case-series records include one variable descriptive statistics.

2.2   CROSS-SECTIONAL STUDIES

A cross-sectional study collects data on a group of subjects at some fixed time, such as all in-patients (census) in a mental health institute and prevalence morbidity survey in a defined community.

2.2.1 HOSPITAL IN-PATIENTS CENSUS

2.2.1.1 OBSERVATIONAL UNITS

The observational units for in-patients census are all the in-patients in a mental hospital/psychiatric unit on a particular day (say July 1 of the year).

2.2.1.2 VARIABLES

The variables to be included in such studies depend on the type of hospital/ unit. However, it is necessary to include important variables such as age, sex, diagnosis, mode of admission status (voluntary, certified, observational, criminal record), and duration of stay in the hospital.

2.2.1.3 RECORD FORM

The record form includes the identification of particulars such as ward, admission number, and initials of the patient.

It is necessary to conduct in-patient census in mental health institute (hospital). The data analysis consists of descriptive statistics according to duration of stay.

2.2.2 MENTAL MORBIDITY STUDIES

2.2.2.1 OBSERVATIONAL UNITS

In prevalence morbidity studies, the sampling unit is the family, and the observational units are all the persons including psychiatric cases in the selected families.

2.2.2.2 VARIABLES

The variables to be studied are specified in the record form/schedules used for the survey. Four schedules are prepared to collect the data.

2.2.2.3 HOUSEHOLD INFORMATION SCHEDULE

This records the data connected with family structure, family size, age of each member of the family, their marital status, education, housing, and identification of the family.

2.2.2.4 SOCIO-ECONOMIC STATUS SCHEDULE

This is used to determine socio-economic status (SES) of each family. The schedule developed by Pareek and Trivedi is standardized for use in rural areas of India. The schedule developed by Kuppuswamy is used for urban sectors.

2.2.2.5 CASE DETECTION SCHEDULE

This contains questions that lead to the identification of all possible mental illness. The sensitivity and specificity of the screening scale to be used in the field settings has to be assessed before using it. The Indian Psychiatric-Survey Schedule (IPSS) prepared by Kapur et al., and the rapid psychiatric examination schedule (RPES) prepared by Sharma are the ones that are most commonly used.

2.2.2.6 CASE RECORD SCHEDULE

This gives all relevant information about the case detected through the case detection schedule and records the findings of examination and final diagnosis. For an operational definition of a case, ICD-11 can be taken as a model.The statistical methods in mental morbidity studies include the prevalence rates for all the major diagnostics categories according to important variables included in the study.

2.3 LONGITUDINAL STUDIES

2.3.1 RETROSPECTIVE STUDIES

Schematic representation of retrospective study design is given in Figure 2.1

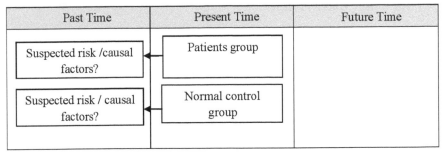

Past Time	Present Time	Future Time
Suspected risk /causal factors? ←	Patients group	
Suspected risk / causal factors? ←	Normal control group	

FIGURE 2.1   Schematic representation of retrospective study design.

The cases in retrospective studies (case-control studies) are individuals selected on the basis of some disease/disorder, and the controls are subjects without the disease/disorder. The history of previous events of both cases and controls are analyzed in an attempt to identify a characteristic or risk factor present in the cases histories but not in the controls histories.

2.3.1.1   PATIENT GROUP AND NORMAL CONTROL GROUP

The investigator sometimes uses matching to associate controls with cases on characteristics such as age, sex, social, and economic status. If an investigator feels that some characteristics are so important that an imbalance between the two groups of patients would affect any conclusion, then he should employ matching. This process ensures that groups will be similar with respect to important characteristics that may otherwise cloud or confound the conclusion. Sometimes, it is recommended to use of the following two controls: one control group similar in some way to the case (e.g., having been hospitalized during the same period of time) and the other control group of healthy subjects.

2.3.1.2   SUSPECTED RISK/CAUSAL FACTORS

These are the factors associated with the psychiatric disorders including genetic, environmental,and so on.

2.3.1.3   RECORD FORM

A typical record form is as given below:

Patient /subject number	Disease/ (present/absent)	age	sex	SES	-	Suspected risk/causal factor (present/absent)
1						
2						
-						

The results of a retrospective study may point to the existence of a real association between a disease and some etiological factor, but they can never prove cause-and-effect relationship. The case-control studies are especially appropriate for studying disease or events, which develop over a long time, and for investigating a preliminary hypothesis. They are generally the quickest and least-expensive studies to understand and are ideal for investigators who need to obtain some preliminary data before writing a proposal for a more complete, expensive, and time-consuming studies. In case-control studies, an estimate of relative risk known as odds ratio (OR) is calculated.

2.3.2 PROSPECTIVE STUDIES

The prospective studies (cohort studies, incidence studies, follow-up studies) select two groups based on exposure. A cohort is a group of people who have something in common and who remain part of a group over an extended time. In medicine, the subjects in cohort studies are selected by some defining characteristic to suspect of being a precursor to or risk factor for a disease. Schematic representation of prospective study design is given in Figure 2.2.

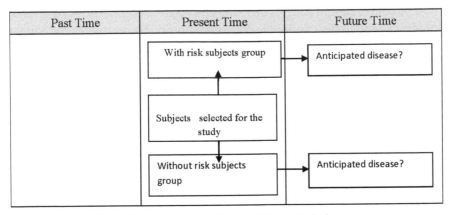

FIGURE 2.2   Schematic representation of prospective study design.

2.3.2.1   WITH RISK SUBJECTS AND WITHOUT RISK SUBJECTS

Researchers select subjects at the onset of the studies and then determine whether they have the risk factor or have been exposed. All subjects are followed over a certain period to observe the effect of the risk factor or exposure (the anticipated disease).

2.3.2.2   ANTICIPATED DISEASE

The anticipated disease/disorder may be any of the mental and behavioral disorder.

2.3.2.3   RECORD FORM

A typical record form is given below:

Subject number	Risk factor (present/absent)	age	sex	-	Anticipated disease (present/absent)
1	-	-	-	-	-
2	-	-	-	-	-
-	-	-	-	-	-

The cohort design permits absolute and relative comparisons of disease incidence among the exposed and the unexposed. These studies have great value when a precise hypothesis has already been formulated, and it is desirable to obtain clear-cut evidence to support or refute it. When the disease is rare, a prospective study may not be possible because the required minimum number of cases will not be available from the population. They also make it difficult for investigators to argue causation because other events occurring in the intervening period may have affected the outcome. Cohort studies that require a long time to complete are especially vulnerable to problems associated with patient follow-ups, particular patient attrition (patients stop participating in the study), and patients' migration. When the data are in the form of counts, the strength of the correlation between the risk factor and the disease may be expressed as risk ratio (RR).

KEYWORDS

- **Case-series analysis**
- **Case-control studies**
- **In-patients census**
- **NIMHANS**

CHAPTER 3

EXPERIMENTAL STUDIES

CONTENTS

3.1   BASIC ELEMENTS OF EXPERIMENTS

3.1.1   EXPERIMENTAL ERROR

There are experimental errors that include all types of extraneous variation due to intrinsic variability of experimental material, lack of uniformity in the methodology of conducting the experiment, and lack of representation of the sample to the population.

3.1.2   BASIC PRINCIPLES OF EXPERIMENTS

3.1.2.1   REPLICATION

An experimenter resorts to the principle of replication in order to average out the influence of the chance factors on different experimental units.

3.1.2.2   RANDOMIZATION

The experimenter resorts to the principle of randomization to provide a logical basis for validity of the statistical tests of significance.

3.1.2.3   LOCAL CONTROL

The experimenter may resort to the principle of local control to reduce the experimental errors by dividing the heterogeneous experimental material into blocks consisting of homogeneous units.

3.1.3   LABORATORY EXPERIMENTS AND CLINICAL EXPERIMENTS

A laboratory experiment takes place in laboratory where experimental manipulation is facilitated. A clinical study takes place in the settings of clinical medicine. Experimental studies in medicine that involve humans are called clinical trials because their purpose is to draw conclusions about a particular procedure or treatment. Thus, clinical trial is a carefully and ethically designed experiment with the aim of answering some precisely framed question.

3.1.4 THERAPEUTIC TRIALS AND PROPHYLACTIC TRIALS

Therapeutic trials are the test of remedies on a disease or a disorder that is followed whenever some improved technique is reported. Such tests of treatment methods differ little from the regular clinical procedures. The differences seem largely a matter of degree of attention to details of whom to test, how to treat, and how to measure the effect of treatment.

The prophylactic trials attempt to present some diseases from occurring by applying a treatment to susceptible persons before that disease has appeared. These trials in medical practice are more convenient to run when the case load of patients at risk is high, the risk factor is not low, and the time between cause and effect is short. The basic principles of these trials are the same as that of the therapeutic trials. In prophylactic trials, the susceptible people are divided into two groups:one group is given the prophylactic and the other is not (control). These groups are then observed over the same period to see if the protected group suffered a lower incidence of the particular disease than the unprotected. These trials have been carried out particularly in infectious diseases.

3.1.5 UNCONTROLLED AND CONTROLLED TRIALS

Uncontrolled trials are studies in which the investigators experiment with the experimental drug (therapy, procedure), but the treatment is not compared with another treatment, at least not formally. The points to be considered are the treatment, patients group, measurement of outcome, record form, and the data analysis.

Controlled trials are studies in which the experimental drug or procedure is compared with another drug or procedure: sometimes a placebo and sometimes the previously accepted treatment. The purpose of an experiment is to determine whether the intervention (treatment) makes a difference. Studies with controls are much more likely than those without controls to detect whether the difference is due to the experimental treatment or to some other factor. Thus, controlled studies are viewed as having far greater validity in medicine than uncontrolled studies. The common way a trial can be controlled is to have two groups of subjects: one that receives the experimental procedure (experimental group) and the other that receives the placebo or standard procedure (control group). The experimental and control groups should be treated alike in all the ways except for the procedures itself so that any differences between the groups will be done to the procedure and not to other factors.

3.2   PARALLEL CONTROL CLINICAL TRIALS

Schematic representation of parallel control clinical trial design is given in Figure 3.1

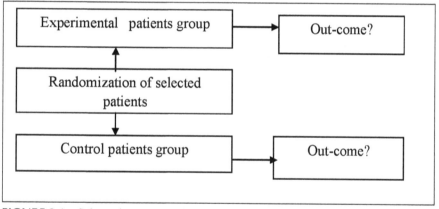

FIGURE 3.1   Schematic representation of parallel control clinical trial design.

3.2.1   TREATMENT AND DISEASE

When a treatment is already in existence, the new form of treatment should normally be compared with the established one. As a first step, the eligible patients from the available patients are selected as per the medical and ethical considerations. After the procedure, a list of volunteers must be short listed. In order to overcome the ethical problem, the volunteers must be informed that they may be assigned to either the experimental or the control group and a written consent of the subjects to participate must be obtained.

3.2.2 EXPERIMENTAL PATIENTS GROUP AND CONTROL PATIENTS GROUP

3.2.2.1 RANDOMIZATION

The volunteers are stratified according to the objectives of the trials. In each group, allot the treatment and controls at random in such a way that the groups are initially equivalent in all respects relevant to the inquiry. The randomized controlled trial is the epitome of all research designs because it provides the strongest evidence for concluding causation. It provides the best insurance that the results were due to the intervention.

3.2.2.2 BLINDING

To reduce the bias, the experimenter may prefer blind trials. In a single-blind study, only the investigator knows of what is administered to each subject. In a double-blind study, neither the subjects nor the investigators know the identity of what is administered.

3.2.3 MODE OF ADMINISTRATION OF THERAPY

In the case of new treatment, the information is at first scanty. The testing may reveal some of the dangers of side effects of the drug. We may choose one dose of a drug out of many and vary the interval of its administration, given it by different routines for different time periods, and so on. Identical procedures should be followed for the control group also.

3.2.4 RECORD FORM

In observing the findings, standard record forms must be drawn up and uniformity in completing must be maintained in both the groups. Every departure from the design of the experiment lowers its efficiency to some extent. The deviations from the procedure laid down may be due to the removal of the patients due to serious side effects, deaths, deterioration of conditions,and so on. These deviations must be considered in the standard analysis of data and valid inferences have to be made.

3.3   FURTHER CONTROL CLINICAL TRIALS

3.3.1   SELF-CONTROL TRIALS

The self-control experimental design (cross-over design) uses two groups of patients: one group is assigned to the experimental treatment and the other group is assigned to the placebo or control treatment. After a time, the experimental treatment and placebo are withdrawn from both groups for a washout period. During the washout period, the patients generally do not receive any treatment. The groups are then given the alternate treatment; that is, the first group now receives the placebo and the second group receives the experimental treatment. Schematic representation of self control trial is given in Figure 3.2

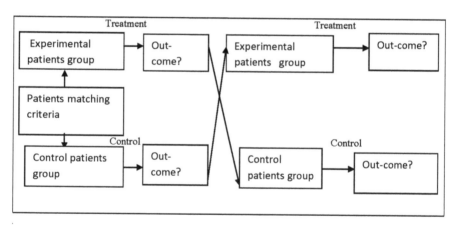

FIGURE 3.2   Schematic representation of self-control clinical trial design.

3.3.2   HISTORICAL CONTROL TRIALS

One can also undertake a cohort study by using information collected in the past and kept in records or files.

Example: We may assess study outcome of 1,000 schizophrenia patients treated with a specific type of psychiatric drug. The existing records may be used to look at improvement of say 1,000 patients who were treated during 2003. This approach to a study is possible if the records on follow-ups are complete and adequately detailed and if the investigator can ascertain the current state of the patients. Schematic representation of historical control trial design is given in Figure 3.3

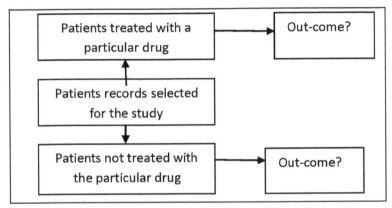

FIGURE 3.3   Schematic representation of historical control study design.

Some investigators call this type of study a historical or retrospective cohort study because historical information is used. That is, events being evaluated actually occurred before the event of the study. Studies that merely describe an investigator's experience with a group of patients and attempt to identify features associated with a good or bad outcome fall under this category.

3.4   INFORMAL DESIGNS OF EXPERIMENTS

The informal designs of experiments are those that normally use a less sophisticated form of analysis to measure the effect of treatment.

3.4.1   BEFORE-AND-AFTER WITHOUT CONTROL GROUP

In this design, a single test group is selected and the dependent variable (DV) is measured before the introduction of the treatment. The treatment is then introduced, and the dependent variable is measured again after the treatment has been introduced. Schematic representation of before-and-after without control group is given in figure 3.4

FIGURE 3.4   Schematic representation of before-and-after without control group design.

The effect of the treatment would be equal to the level of the phenomenon after the treatment minus the level of the phenomenon before the treatment. The main difficulty here is that with the passage of time, considerable extraneous variation may be there in the treatment effect.

3.4.2   AFTER-ONLY WITH CONTROL GROUP

In this experiment design, two groups, experimental group and control group, of patients are selected and the treatment is introduced into the experimental group only. The dependent variable is then measured in both the groups at the same time. Here, the two groups are identical with respect to their behavior toward the phenomenon considered. Schematic representation of after-only with control group is given in figure 3.5

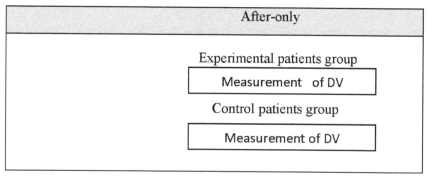

FIGURE 3.5   Schematic representation of after-only with control group design.

The treatment impact is assessed by subtracting the value of the dependent variable in the control group from its value in the experimental group. The advantage of this design is that the data can be collected without introducing problem with the passage of time.

3.4.3   BEFORE-AND-AFTER WITH CONTROL GROUP

In this design, two groups are selected, and the dependent variable is measured in both the groups for an identical time period before the treatment. The treatment is then introduced into the experimental group only, and the dependent variable is measured in both for an identical time period after the introduction of the treatment. Schematic representation of before-and-after with control group is given in figure 3.6

FIGURE 3.6   Schematic representation of before-and-after with control group design.

The treatment effect is determined by subtracting the change in the dependent variable in the control group from the change in the dependent variable in the experimental group. This design avoids extraneous variation resulting both from the passage of time and from noncomparability of the experimental and control groups.

3.5 FORMAL DESIGNS OF EXPERIMENTS

3.5.1 COMPLETELY RANDOMIZED DESIGN

The completely randomized design (CRD) is the simplest of all the experimental designs based on the principles of replication and randomization. Let us suppose that there are k treatments and the ith treatment is being replicated n_i times. In CRD, the whole of the experimental units are distributed completely at random to the treatments subject to the condition that the ith treatment occurs n_i times. Randomization assumes that extraneous factors do not continuously influence one treatment.

Layout: The layout of CRD is as given below:

Treatment 1	Treatment 2	-	Treatment k
x_{11}	x_{21}		x_{k1}
x_{12}	x_{22}		x_{k2}
x_{1n_1}	x_{2n_2}	-	x_{kn_k}

If some of the observations for any treatment are lost, then the standard analysis can be carried out on the available data. The analysis of the data in CRD is analogous to the ANOVA for one-way classification.

3.5.2 RANDOMIZED BLOCK DESIGN

If the whole of the experimental material is not homogenous, then the randomized block design (RBD) is the simple method of controlling the variability of the experimental material. The RBD consists in grouping the experimental material into relatively homogenous strata called blocks, and the treatments are applied at random to the units within each block and replicated over all the blocks. The treatments are allocated at random within the units of each block, and thus randomization is restricted. Thus, if it is desired to control one source of variation by stratification, the experimenter should select RBD rather than CRD.

   Layout The layout of RBD is as given below:

Blocks	Treatment 1	Treatment 2	-	Treatment k
1	x_{11}	x_{21}		x_{k1}
2	x_{12}	x_{22}		x_{k2}
-	.	.		.
r	x_{1r}	x_{2r}	.	x_{kr}

The statistical analysis of data in RBD is analogous to two-way ANOVA.

3.5.3 FACTORIAL DESIGNS

In factorial experiments, the effects of several factors of variation are studied and investigated simultaneously. Here, the treatments are the combinations of different factors under study. In these experiments, an attempt is made to estimate the effects of each of the factors and also their interactive effects. Let us suppose that there are p different doses of diazepam and q different doses of nitrazepam. The p and q are termed as the levels of the factors diazepam and nitrazepam,respectively. A series of experiments in which only one factor is varied at a time would be lengthy, costly, and unsatisfactory because of systematic change in the general background conditions. Moreover, these simple experiments do not tell us anything about the interaction effect. Alternatively, we try to investigate the variation in several factors simultaneously by conducting a $p \times q$ factorial experiment. In general, if the levels of various factors are equal, then r^s experiment means a factorial experiment with s factors each at r levels.

3.5.3.1 2²-FACTORIAL DESIGN

In 2^2 (or 2×2) factorial experiment, we have two factors each at two levels, and hence there are four treatment combinations in all. Let the capital letters A and B indicate the name of the two factors under study. Let the small letters"a" and "b"denote one of the two levels of each of the corresponding factors, and this will be usually called the second level. The first level of A and B are generally expressed by the absence of the corresponding small letter in the treatment combinations. The four treatment combinations may be enumerated as follows:
    1: Both A and B are at the first level

a: A is at second level and B is at the first level
b: A is at first level and B is at the second level
ab: Both A and B are at the second level

Layout: The layout of 2^2-factorial design with RBD is given below:

Blocks	Treatments			
	1	**a**	**b**	**ab**
1	x_{11}	x_{21}	x_{31}	x_{41}
2	x_{12}	x_{22}	x_{32}	x_{42}
-				
r	x_{1r}	x_{2r}	x_{3r}	x_{4r}
Total	(1)	(a)	(b)	(ab)

3.5.4 ANALYSIS OF COVARIANCE DESIGN

In analysis of covariance (ANCOVA), it is assumed that the observed values (y) are attributed to the treatments applied and not to any other causal circumstances. Sometimes, some concomitant variable (x) is correlated with the dependent variable (y). The marks scored in psychiatry by a group of multipurpose health workers after conducting a training program may be related to the marks scored by the group before conducting the training program. In such situations, the researcher should use the statistical technique of ANCOVA for valid comparison of treatment effects.

Layout: The layout of the ANCOVA design is as given below:

Treatment 1		Treatment 2			Treatment k	
x	y	x	y	-	x	y
x_{11}	y_{11}	x_{21}	y_{21}		x_{k1}	y_{k1}
x_{12}	y_{12}	x_{22}	y_{22}		x_{k2}	y_{k2}
- -		- -		-	- -	
x_{1n_1}	y_{1n_1}	x_{2n_2}	y_{2n_2}	-	x_{kn_k}	y_{kn_k}

3.5.5 REPEATED MEASURES DESIGN

The repeated measures design (also known as within-subject design) uses the same subjects with every condition of the research. For instance, repeated measures are collected in a longitudinal study in which change over time is assessed.

Layout: The layout of the design is as given below:

Subject	Repeat 1	Repeat 2	-	Repeat k
1	x_{11}	x_{21}		x_{k1}
2	x_{12}	x_{22}		x_{k2}
-	-	-	-	-
n	x_{1n}	x_{2n}		x_{kn}

One disadvantage to the repeated measures design is that it may not be possible for each participant to be present in all conditions of the experiment, especially severely diseased subjects tend to drop out of a longitudinal study. Removing these subjects would bias the design.

KEYWORDS

- ANCOVA
- Clinical trials
- Experimental errors

CHAPTER 4

ONE-VARIABLE DESCRIPTIVE STATISTICS

CONTENTS

4.1   CLASSIFICATION AND TABULATION OF DATA

The observations on each variable have to be classified and presented in the form of tables. The main objectives of classification are to simplify the complex nature of the data, tailoring it up, and make it easy to grasp. The classification by person may be made according to qualitative and quantitative aspects.

4.1.1   QUALITATIVE VARIABLE DATA

In the classification of a qualitative variable data, a natural classification system may be available. For example, in the classification of patients according to sex, it is enough if we count the number of males and the number of females. The classified data have to be presented in the form of tables separately for each variable or for groups of variables. The total of the frequencies and the relative frequencies in the table will aid in the interpretation of the results. Appropriate title must be given at the top of the table. The source of data and the new terms used must be specified at the bottom of the table. For example, the sex distribution of the 40 registered psychiatric patients (data in Appendix I) is as given in Table 4.1.

TABLE 4.1   Sex distribution of 40 psychiatric patients

Sex	Frequency
Males	24
Females	16
Total	40

4.1.2   QUANTITATIVE VARIABLE DATA

4.1.2.1   ARRAY

The first step in the classification of a quantitative variable data is to arrange the raw data in an array of ascending or descending order.

Example: The array of the 40 registered patients (data in Appendix I) according to age is as given below:

4	9	10	11	12	12	13	16	19	21
22	23	24	24	25	25	25	26	26	27
27	29	29	30	31	33	35	35	40	44
48	50	51	58	60	60	65	68	76	80

4.1.2.2 CLASSIFICATION

In the classification of the quantitative variable data, the optimum number and length of frequency classes depend on the size, nature of the data, and the purpose of the study. Generally, the frequency classes are of equal size, mutually exclusive, and exhaustive. The main purpose of classification of quantitative variable data is to determine the nature of the frequency distribution: normal, uniform, exponential, etc.

Example: The age distribution of the 40 registered patients is as given in Table 4.2.

TABLE 4.2   Age distribution of 40 psychiatric patients

Age	Frequencies
Below 10	2
10–19	7
20–29	14
30–39	5
40–49	3
50–59	3
60–69	3
70–79	2
80–89	1
Total	40

This age distribution follows approximate normal distribution. The frequency distribution of age increases up to 20–29 age group and decreases thereafter.

4.2 GRAPHICAL REPRESENTATION OF CLASSIFIED DATA

In more complex situation of presentation, further to see the shape and pattern of frequency distribution, graphs and diagrams may be used with or without the frequency tables. They are good visual and mental aids for both professionals and laymen. Generally, the graphs are drawn for quantitative variable data and diagrams are drawn for qualitative variable data.

4.2.1 QUALITATIVE VARIABLE DATA

4.2.1.1 BAR DIAGRAM

In bar diagram, on a common base line, vertical or horizontal bars are drawn with their heights proportional to the frequencies. The bars are of equal width and successive bars are drawn at equal distances. Composite, component, or percentage bar diagrams may be drawn depending on the size and nature of the classified data. This diagram is especially preferred for discrete data.

Example: The bar diagram showing the age distributions of 10 years' duration of the 40 psychiatric patients of NIMHANS hospital (data in Appendix I) is shown as bar diagram (Figure 4.1).

FIGURE 4.1   Bar diagram showing the age distribution of 40 psychiatric patients.

4.2.2   QUANTITATIVE VARIABLE DATA

4.2.2.1   FREQUENCY POLYGON

In frequency polygon, the frequencies are plotted on a graph sheet, and the lines joining these points are drawn. More than one frequency polygon may be drawn on the same graph sheet, and thus several frequency distributions may be compared. This graphical representation is more appropriate for continuous data as shown in Figure 4.2. It can be viewed that the psychiatric patients of young age groups and old-age groups in the community are under-represented at NIMHANS hospital.

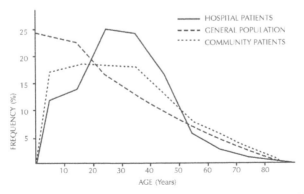

FIGURE 4.2   Frequency polygons showing age distributions of 500 psychiatric patients.

4.2.2.2 HISTOGRAM

In histogram, on a common base line, rectangles are drawn with their areas proportional to the frequencies. These rectangles are in juxtaposition, and there will be no gaps between them. This diagram is more appropriate for data in ratio scale of measurement and especially when the frequency classes are of unequal widths as shown in Figure 4.3. In order to draw this diagram, the frequencies of the classes of varying duration of illness had to be converted into frequencies for unit duration of illness.

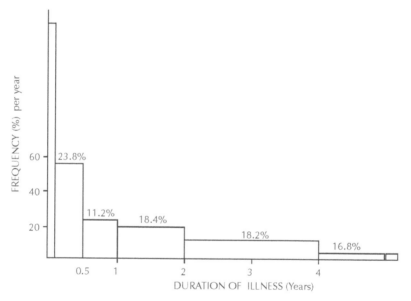

FIGURE 4.3   Histogram showing the duration of illness of 500 psychiatric patients.

4.3   SUMMARIZING DATA: AVERAGES

The summarization figures of measurement of characteristics of frequency distribution will be helpful to understand the data more clearly. The observed values of a psychiatric variable are not equal, but we can notice a general tendency of these values to cluster around a particular value. It is convenient to characterize and represent each group of observations by such a value that is called the central tendency or the average of that group.

4.3.1 QUANTITATIVE VARIABLE DATA

4.3.1.1 MEAN

The mean (arithmetic mean) is obtained by dividing the sum of observations by the total number of observations. Therefore,

$$\text{Mean} = \frac{\text{Sum of observations}}{\text{Total number of observations}}$$

Symbolically,

$$\bar{x} = \frac{1}{n}\sum x_i$$

where x_i are the observed values and n is the number of observations.

The population mean is denoted by μ, and the sample mean is denoted by $\bar{x}$. The mean is sensitive to the presence of extreme values in the data, and hence it does not give fair idea of central tendency when the extreme values or outliers are present in the data.

4.3.1.2 MEDIAN

The median is the middle most value of the observations arranged in an ascending or descending order of magnitude. It divides the distribution into two equal parts, and hence it is a position value.

4.3.1.3 MODE

The mode is that value of the observations, which occurs most frequently. There may be more than one mode in a frequency distribution.

Example: Let us suppose that the marks scored in a test (out of 10) by a group of five students are given by 7, 4, 1, 3, and 5. For this data,

Array:	1, 3, 4, 5, 7
Sample size (n):	5
Sum of observations: (Σx)	20
Mean ($\bar{x}$):	4.0
Median:	4
Mode:	not available

4.3.2 QUALITATIVE VARIABLE DATA

4.3.2.1 PROPORTION AND PERCENTAGE

A proportion of a category of a qualitative variable is given by
$$P = \text{numerator/denominator}$$

A percentage is defined as follows

$$\text{Percentage, (\%)} = \text{proportion} \times 100$$
$$= p \times 100$$

Thus, the percentages of frequencies of a categorical variable (qualitative variable) add to 100, and the proportions of the frequencies add to 1.

Example: The proportions and percentages of males and females of the 40 registered patients (data in Appendix I) are given in the following table:

Sex	Frequency	Proportion	Percentage
Male	24	0.6	60.0
Female	16	0.4	40.0
Total	40	1.0	100.0

4.3.2.2 RATE AND RATIO

A rate measures diseases, disabilities, and injuries per unit population. That is,

$$\text{Rate} = \frac{\text{Numerator} \times \text{duration of time} \times \text{k}}{\text{Denominator}}$$

$$= \frac{\text{Number infected} \times \text{duration of time} \times k}{\text{Population at risk}}$$

When the denominator consists of all those who have the chance of getting the disease, it is known as the population at risk.

Example: There are 11 admissions for in-patients services out of a total of 40 registered patients. Then,

$$\text{Rate of admission} = \frac{11 \times 100}{40} = 27.5\%$$

The rates may be crude (crude birth rate), specific (sex specific rate), or standardized (standardized death rate).

A ratio is defined as follows:

$$\text{Ratio} = \frac{\text{Numerator} \times \text{point of time} \times k}{\text{Denominator}}$$

$$= \frac{\text{Number infected} \times \text{point of time} \times 1000}{\text{Population at Risk}}$$

Thus, in a ratio, the numerator and the denominator are independent. A rate refers to a period of time, whereas a ratio refers to a point of time. For examples, the sex ratio of Indian population is 940 females per 1,000 males.

4.3.2.3   INDICATORS AND INDEX

An indicator can be defined as something that helps us understand what we are, where we are going, and how far we are from the goal. Therefore, it can be a number or a graphic. Health indicators are established to monitor the health status of a given population and to evaluate the number of individuals affected by a particular disease within a given time period and the total number of cases of that disease. It is also used to evaluate health risks and performance of health system. An index is a statistic giving the value of a quantity such as cost per day per patient, etc., relative to its level at some fixed time or place, which conventionally is given the number hundred.

4.4　SUMMARIZING DATA: DISPERSION

The observed values of a variable tend to spread over an interval rather than cluster closely around the central average. The characteristics of the scatter or spread of the observed values in the neighborhood of the central average is called dispersion.

4.4.1　QUANTITATIVE VARIABLE DATA

4.4.1.1　RANGE

The minimum value, the maximum value, and the range of observed values of a variable are the crude measures of dispersion. The range is given by

$$R = X_{maximum} - X_{minimum}$$

4.4.1.2　STANDARD DEVIATION

The range depends only on the extreme values, and it does not deal with the variation within the group. The standard deviation is the root-mean-squared deviation measured from the mean. The population standard deviation is denoted by σ and that of the sample by S (or SD). Thus,

$$S = \sqrt{\frac{1}{n}\sum\left(x - \bar{x}\right)^2}$$

4.4.1.3　COEFFICIENT OF VARIATION

The coefficient of variation (CV) is a relative measure of dispersion. It is given by the following relation:

$$CV = \frac{Standard\ deviation \times 100}{Mean}$$

Example: Let us suppose that the marks scored in a test by a group of five students are given by 7, 4, 1, 3, and 5. For this data,

Minimum value = 1

Maximum value = 7

Range = 7 − 1 = 6

To calculate standard deviation, the computation table is given below:

Student	x	$(x - \bar{x})$	$(x - \bar{x})^2$
1	7	3	9
2	4	0	0
3	1	−3	9
4	3	−1	1
5	5	1	1
Total	20	0	20
Mean	4.0	0	-

Now, the standard deviation is calculated as follows:

$$S = \sqrt{\frac{20}{5}} = \sqrt{4} = 2.0$$

The coefficient of variation is calculated as follows:

$$CV = \frac{2 \times 100}{4} = 50\%$$

4.4.2   QUALITATIVE VARIABLE DATA

4.4.2.1   FREQUENCY DISTRIBUTION

The frequency distribution and the relative frequency distribution serve as the measurement of dispersion in case of qualitative variable data. For example, the diagnostic distribution of the 40 registered patients (data in Appendix I) is as given in Table 4.3.

TABLE 4.3 Diagnostic distribution of 40 psychiatric patients

Disorder	Number of patients	(%)
1. Organic psychosis	2	5.0
2. Substance use disorder	1	2.5
3. Schizophrenia	8	20.0
4. Mania	-	-
5. Bipolar affective disorder	8	20.0
6. Endogenous depression	7	17.5
7. Phobia	-	-
8. Obsessive compulsive neuroses	2	5.0
9. Anxiety neurosis	1	2.5
10. Neurotic depression	2	5.0
11. Dissociative disorder	2	5.0
12. Somatoform disorder	-	-
13. Behavioral syndrome	-	-
14. Personality disorder	-	-
15. Mental retardation	2	5.0
16. Developmental disorder	4	10.0
17. Behavior/emotional disorder	1	2.5
18. Epilepsy	-	-
All disorders	40	100.0

4.5 SUMMARIZING DATA: SKEWNESS AND KURTOSIS

4.5.1 SKEWNESS

The skewness is the lack of symmetry. A perfectly bell-shaped curve has no skewness. Hence, a distribution is skew if the mean, median, and mode do not have the same value. The skewness may be positive such as age distribution of dissociative disorder patients (CON), negative such as age distribution of somatoform (SOM) disorder patients, or zero such as age distribution of obsessive and compulsive disorder (OCD) patients at NIM-HANS hospital as shown in Figure 4.4.

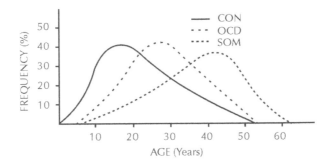

FIGURE 4.4 Frequency curves showing positively skewed, negatively skewed, and symmetrical distributions.

4.5.1.1 COEFFICIENT OF SKEWNESS

One of the measures of skewness is coefficient of skewness that usually lies between -1 and 1. It is given by

$$\text{Coefficient of skewness} = \frac{\text{Mean} - \text{Mode}}{\text{Standard deviation}}$$

4.5.2 KURTOSIS

Kurtosis is the measure of the relative flatness of the top of the frequency curve. A frequency curve may be symmetrical, but it may fail to have peakedness as that of a normal curve. The frequency distribution may have the same variability, but this may be more or less peaked than that of the normal curve. The kurtosis may be classified as mesokurtic (medium kurtosis), leptokurtic (high kurtosis), and platykurtic (low kurtosis) as shown in Figure 4.5, where obsessive thought disorder (OTD), obsessive compulsive disorders (OCD), dissociative disorder and somatoform disorder (DSD) at NIMHANS hospital.

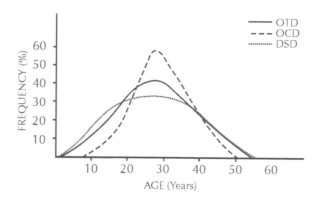

FIGURE 4.5   Frequency curves showing leptokurtic, mesokurtic, and platykurtic distributions.

4.6   DESCRIPTIVE STATISTICS FOR SPATIAL DATA

4.6.1   CLASSIFICATION OF SPATIAL DATA

The geographical data are sometimes arranged alphabetically. The spatial characteristic of the data when presented in tables is largely obscured. It is advantageous to incorporate both the geographical and political aspects in maps.

4.6.2   SPOT MAPS

The maps provide the necessary medium for presenting real relationship of spatial data clearly, meaningfully, and adequately. Maps are often indispensible in locating problems, analyzing data, and discovering hidden facts and relationships. It is advantageous to incorporate both the geographical and political aspects in maps. The geographical aspect is important to determine the causal factors of disorders/diseases. The political aspect is important for effective mental health delivery systems. There are spot maps, shaded maps, and superimposed maps. In spot maps, the size of the symbol may be proportional to the magnitude of the phenomena represented. Symbols may be in the form of circles. The area of the circle may be proportional to the value represented.

Example: The 36 government mental hospitals in India are presented as spot map as shown in Figure 4.6.

FIGURE 4.6   Spot map portraying bed occupancies in government mental hospitals in India.

The geographical area that is too far to a government mental hospital in India may be located using the spot map.

4.6.3 DENSITY OF PATIENTS

It is given by

$$\text{Density of patients} = \frac{\text{Total number of patients}}{\text{Area in square kilometers}}$$

Example: The density of psychiatric patients in India is calculated as follows:

$$\text{Density of patients} = \frac{7,20,00000}{33,00000} = 21.8 \text{ per square kilometer}$$

4.7   DESCRIPTIVE STATISTICS FOR TIME-RELATED DATA

4.7.1   CLASSIFICATION OF TIME-RELATED DATA

The classification of time period depends on the purpose of the epidemiological study and the time series analysis required for the purpose. The classification can be made according to hours, days, weeks, months, years, etc., depending on the purpose of the study.

4.7.2   EPIDEMIOLOGICAL CURVES

An epidemic curve is defined as a plot of the number of cases against time of onset of disease, with time on the horizontal -axis, and the number of new cases on the vertical -axis. It is a method of visualizing the progression of a disease over time, which helps epidemiologists to answer several important questions.

4.7.3   EXPECTATION OF DURATION OF TIME AND TIME SERIES COMPONENTS

The expectation of duration of time (Life tables) and Time series components (Trend, seasonal variation, cyclic components) are important statistical methods relating to time (Chapter 14).

KEYWORDS

- **Coefficient of variation**
- **Descriptive statistics**
- **Quantitative/qualitative variable data**

CHAPTER 5

MENTAL HEALTH STATISTICS

CONTENTS

5.1   DEMOGRAPHIC INDICATORS

Demography is the study of the composition, distribution, and growth of human population, and their interrelationships with social, economic, and behavioral factors. In addition to statistics relating to existing mental health conditions and available mental health care facilities, knowledge of demographic indicators is important for psychiatric service and research for specification of goals and targets in terms of measurable outputs.

5.1.1   POPULATION SIZE

Population size is an important figure as it is utilized in deriving various mental morbidity indices.

5.1.1.1   MALTHUS THEORY

This theory states that the human population will expand exponentially, whereas the means of subsistence will increase more slowly, with the consequence that ultimately the size will be kept in check by famine, disease (including mental disorders), and war.

5.1.2   POPULATION COMPOSITION

5.1.2.1   AGE DISTRIBUTION

Age distribution of the population provides the true picture regarding the risk of various mental and behavioral disorders associated with different age groups.

5.1.2.2   SEX DISTRIBUTION

Sex distribution of the population will help in studying different mental and behavioral disorders associated with each sex. This is important for improving the mental health care of the entire population.

5.1.2.3 DOMICILE DISTRIBUTION

The domicile (rural–urban) distribution of the population will help in preparing the required mental health programs for these sectors separately.

5.1.2.4 RELIGION/CASTE DISTRIBUTIONS

Most of the psychiatric disorders are associated with religion/caste distributions.

5.1.2.5 FAMILY SIZE

The average family size is also important since it varies with several psychiatric disorders.

5.1.3 POPULATION DISTRIBUTION

The population distribution of a geographical region can be studied by calculating the density of population.

5.1.3.1 DENSITY OF POPULATION

The density of population per square kilometer of a given geographical region is given by the following relation:

$$\text{Density of population} = \frac{\text{Total population of the area}}{\text{Area in Square kilometers}}$$

The density of population in urban locality may be calculated as per persons per room to determine overcrowding.

5.1.4 POPULATION GROWTH

The growth rate of population in a given geographical region is studied by calculating the growth rate of population.

5.1.4.1 ANNUAL GROWTH RATE OF POPULATION

It is given by the following relation:

$$\text{Annual growth rate} = \frac{\text{Increase / decrease in population during the year} \times 1000}{\text{Population as on 1 July of the year}}$$

5.1.5 MEASURES OF FERTILITY AND MORTALITY

A knowledge of the rates of fertility and mortality in a community is important for planning mental health facilities and services for various groups of people.

5.1.5.1 CRUDE BIRTH RATE

The annual crude birth rate (CBR) is the general rate of fertility. It is defined as follows:

$$\text{CBR} = \frac{\text{Number of live births during the year} \times 1000}{\text{Population as on July 1 of the year}}$$

5.1.5.2 CRUDE DEATH RATE

The annual crude death rate (CDR) is the general rate of mortality. It is defined as follows:

$$\text{CDR} = \frac{\text{Number of deaths during the year} \times 1000}{\text{Population as on July 1 of the year}}$$

5.2 DEMOGRAPHIC INDICATORS OF INDIA

The demographic indicators of India for the year 2012 are in Table 5.1.

TABLE 5.1   Demographic indicators of India

1. Population size (in crores)		123
2. Age distribution (%):	0–9	19.6
	10–19	18.7
	20–29	19.4
	30–39	14.4
	40–49	11.6
	50–59	8.1
	60–69	5.0
	70–79	2.4
	80–	0.8
3. Sex distribution (%):	Male	51.5
	Female	48.5
4. Domicile distributions (%):	Rural	68.8
	Urban	31.2
5. Religion distribution (%):	Hindu	80.5
	Muslim	13.4
	Christian	2.3
	All others	3.8
6. Average family size		4.8
7. Densityof population (per square kilometer)		382
8. Annual growth rate (%)		1.4
9. Crude birth rate		20.6
10. Crude death rate		7.4

5.3   MEASURES OF MENTAL MORBIDITY

The prevalence rates and the incidence rates are the important indices to measure epidemiological situation, suggest priorities, and assess the progress made in the control of diseases/disorders.

5.3.1 PREVALENCE RATE

The prevalence rate (point) is the rate at which people having the disease at a particular point of time. That is,

$$\text{Prevalence rate} = \frac{\text{Number of cases at a particular point of time} \times 1000}{\text{Population at risk at the particular point of time}}$$

The prevalence rates are determined for chronic illnesses such as mental and behavioral disorders. The lack of absolute standard criteria for defining a case is the foremost among the methodological problems in psychiatric epidemiological field.

5.3.2 INCIDENCE RATE

The incidence rate is the rate at which people without the disease develop the disease during a specified period of time (say 1year). That is,

$$\text{Incidence rate} = \frac{\text{Number of new cases during the period} \times 1000}{\text{Population at risk during the period}}$$

The incidence rates are usually determined for acute diseases such as infectious diseases, as their onsets are sharply defined. However, in community psychiatry, these rates are also important to answer the question of whether the growth of urbanization leads to increase in mental stress and hence mental disorders.

5.4 MENTAL MORBIDITY IN INDIA

5.4.1 PREVALENCE RATES AND INCIDENCE RATES

The prevalence rate of mental and behavioral disorders in India is estimated to be 58.2 per 1,000 population. The annual incidence rate of mental and behavioral disorders in India is estimated to be 17.1 per 1,000 population. The details are given in Table 5.2.

TABLE 5.2 Prevalence rates and incidence rates of mental and behavior disorders

Disorders	Prevalence rate	Annual incidence rate
1. Organic psychosis	0.4	0.6
2. Substance use disorder	6.9	0.1
3. Schizophrenia	2.7	1.2
4. Mania	0.7	0.1
5.Bipolar affective disorder	2.7	0.9
6. Endogenous depression	8.9	5.4
7. Phobia	4.2	1.8
8. Obsessive compulsive disorder	3.1	0.3
9. Anxiety neurosis	5.8	1.8
10. Neurotic depression	3.1	1.2
11.Dissociative disorder	4.5	1.5
12. Somatoform disorder	0.6	0.9
13. Behavioral syndrome	0.1	0.1
14. Personality disorder	0.5	0.1
15. Mental retardation	6.8	0.3
16. Developmental disorder	0.1	0.1
17. Behavioral/emotional disorder	2.7	0.6
18. Epilepsy	4.4	0.1
All disorders	58.2	17.1

5.4.2 AGE-WISE PREVALENCE RATES

Age-wise prevalence rates of mental and behavioral disorders in India are given in Table 5.3

TABLE 5.3 Age-wise prevalence rates of mental and behavioral disorders in India (rate per 1,000 population)

	Disorder	Combined	0–9	10–19	20–29	30–39	40–49	50–59	60–69	70–79	80–
1	Organic psychosis	0.4	–	–	–	0.2	0.6	1.3	2.0	2.6	**4.1**
2	Substance use disorder	6.9	–	1.9	4.5	8.1	15.9	**20.6**	15.4	6.3	-
3	Schizophrenia	2.7	–	1.1	4.3	**5.6**	5.2	3.6	1.1	–	–
4	Mania	0.7	–	0.2	1.0	**2.0**	1.7	0.5	–	–	–
5	Bipolar affective disorder	2.7	–	–	2.5	6.1	**7.4**	4.2	3.0	2.1	1.9
6	Endogenous Depression	8.9	–	0.4	4.9	11.7	17.2	21.7	27.7	32.0	**33.7**
7	Phobic neurosis	4.2	3.7	**12.7**	5.9	–	–	–	–	–	–
8	Anxiety neurosis	5.8	2.2	6.4	7.5	**8.9**	6.0	4.4	3.0	0.6	–
9	Obsessive Compulsive neurosis	3.1	–	1.3	**7.0**	6.5	4.2	0.9	–	–	–
10	Neurotic depression	3.1	–	1.4	3.6	5.1	**6.2**	5.2	4.8	3.2	–
11	Dissociative disorder	4.5	–	0.1	5.5	**10.8**	9.7	8.0	2.0	–	–
12	Somatoform disorder	0.6	–	0.1	0.3	0.8	1.6	**1.8**	1.3	1.0	0.6
13	Behavioral syndrome	0.1	–	–	0.1	**0.3**	0.1	–	–	–	–
14	Personality disorder	0.5	–	–	0.7	**2.0**	0.7	–	–	–	–
15	Mental retardation	6.8	**14.4**	12.9	5.8	2.7	0.4	–	–	–	–
16	Developmental disorder	0.1	**0.3**	0.2	–	–	–	–	–	–	–
17	Behavioral/emotional disorder	2.7	3.3	**7.4**	3.4	–	–	–	–	–	–
18	Epilepsy	4.4	4.8	**7.1**	5.7	5.0	2.1	0.4	–	–	–
	All disorders	58.2	28.7	53.2	62.7	75.8	**79.0**	72.6	60.3	47.8	40.3

5.4.2.1   REMARKS

It can be noted that in psychiatric patient population, the prevalence rates increase with age exponentially in respect of organic psychosis and endogenous depression. The prevalence rates are highest in the youngest age groups and decrease gradually in respect of mental retardation and developmental disorders. In the remaining diagnostic categories, the distributions are asymptotic normal.

5.4.3   SEX-WISE PREVALENCE RATES

Sex-wise prevalence rates of mental and behavioral disorders in India is given in Table 5.4

TABLE 5.4   Sex-wise prevalence rates of mental and behavioral disorders in India

Disorders	Combined	Male	Female
1. Organic psychosis	0.4	0.2	0.6
2. Substance use disorder	6.9	11.9	1.7
3. Schizophrenia	2.7	2.3	3.2
4. Mania	0.7	1.2	0.1
5. Bipolar affective disorder	2.7	2.3	3.2
6. Endogenous depression	8.9	5.6	12.3
7. Phobia	4.2	2.4	6.0
8. Obsessive compulsive disorder	3.1	1.7	4.6
9. Anxiety neurosis	5.8	3.2	8.4
10. Neurotic depression	3.1	1.2	5.2
11. Dissociative disorder	4.5	1.2	8.0
12. Somatoform disorder	0.6	0.7	0.4
13. Behavioral syndrome	0.1	0.1	0.1
14. Personality disorder	0.5	1.0	0.2
15. Mental retardation	6.8	9.1	4.4
16. Developmental disorder	0.1	0.1	0.1
17. Behavioral/emotional disorder	2.7	2.7	2.7
18. Epilepsy	4.4	4.9	3.9
All disorders	58.2	51.9	64.8

5.4.3.1   REMARKS

The prevalence rate was 51.9 for males and 64.8 for females. Manic affective psychosis, mental retardation, alcohol/drug addiction, and personality disorders were significantly high in males, whereas organic psychosis, endogenous depression, and all neurotic disorders were significantly high among females.

5.4.4   DOMICILE-WISE PREVALENCE RATES

Domicile wise-prevalence rates of mental and behavioral disorders in India are given in Table 5.5

TABLE 5.5   Domicile wise-prevalence rates of mental and behavioral disorders in India

Disorders	Combined	Rural	Urban
1. Organic psychosis	0.4	0.6	0.1
2. Substance use disorder	6.9	7.3	5.8
3. Schizophrenia	2.7	2.6	2.9
4. Mania	0.7	0.6	0.8
5.Bipolar affective disorder	2.7	2.7	3.0
6. Endogenous depression	8.9	7.7	14.1
7. Phobia	4.2	2.4	8.0
8. Obsessive compulsive disorder	3.1	2.3	5.0
9. Anxiety neurosis	5.8	3.1	11.6
10. Neurotic depression	3.1	1.1	7.7
11.Dissociative disorder	4.5	5.0	3.4
12. Somatoform disorder	0.6	0.8	0.2
13. Behavioral syndrome	0.1	0.1	0.1
14. Personality disorder	0.5	0.5	0.7
15. Mental retardation	6.8	6.3	8.8
16. Developmental disorder	0.1	0.1	0.1
17. Behavioral/emotional disorder	2.7	1.0	5.9
18. Epilepsy	4.4	4.8	2.5
All disorders	58.2	48.9	80.6

5.4.4.1 REMARKS

The prevalence rate was 48.9 for rural sectors and 80.6 for urban sectors. Only epilepsy and hysteria were significantly high in rural communities, whereas endogenous depression, mental retardation, all neurotic disorders (except hysteria), and behavioral/emotional disorders were significantly high in urban communities.

5.5 MENTAL HEALTH DELIVERY SYSTEMS IN INDIA

5.5.1 CLASSIFICATION

A broad classification of mental health delivery systems in India is as given below:
1. Mental Health Institutes (Hospitals)
    (a) State government mental hospitals
    (b) Central government mental hospitals
    (c) Autonomous body hospitals
    (d) Private hospitals
2. Psychiatric Rehabilitation Centers
3. Hospital Psychiatric Units
    (a) Medical college hospital psychiatric units
    (b) District hospital psychiatric units
    (c) Specialized hospital psychiatric units
4. Psychiatry Clinics
5. Prison Psychiatric Services
6. Community Mental Health Delivery Systems
    (a) Satellite clinics
    (b) Mental morbidity studies
    (c) Indian system of medicine

5.6 MENTAL HEALTH SERVICE INDICATORS

5.6.1 OUT-PATIENT SERVICE INDICATORS (YEAR)

The out-patients service indicators are common for all mental health delivery systems irrespective of whether in-patients service is available or not. These indicators refer to a particular time period usually 1year, and the data collected are subjected to case-series analysis. The out-patients population forms two sub-populations: newly registered patients and the follow-up patients. The important indicators are

1. Number of new registrations (year)
2. Age distribution
3. Sex distribution
4. Diagnostic distribution
5. Rate of follow-up attendance

$$\text{Rate of follow-up attendance} = \frac{\text{Total follow-up attendance during the year}}{\text{Number of new registrations during the year}}$$

The characteristics of the registered patients are based on the disorders/diseases for which the mental health facilities are being sought, and hence such data may not be a fair representation of the diseases/disorders in the surrounding community. Still they have several administrative and clinical values. Although these data do not provide the estimation at the community level, they are used in spelling out the dimensions of the problems and their applications in planning process and quality-of-life ascertainment. The annual seasonal variation of the disorders in the community may be reflected by changes in the new registrations of the hospital.

5.6.2 ADMITTED PATIENTS (YEAR)

The admitted patients for in-patients treatment form a sub-population of the registered patients. Hence, it is restricted only to mental health institutes (hospitals) and hospital psychiatric units where in-patients facilities are available. Again, these indicators refer to a particular time period (say 1year). The important indicators are the following:

6. Number of admitted patients (year)
7. Rate of admission

$$\text{Rate of admission (\%)} = \frac{\text{Number of patients admitted during the year} \times 100}{\text{Number of new registrations during the year}}$$

5.6.3   IN-PATIENT SERVICE INDICATORS (JULY 1 OF THE YEAR)

The characteristic distributions of in-patients on a particular day (say July 1 of the year) is an important aspect to compare and evaluate the services of a mental health institute (hospital) and hospital psychiatric units. This can be done by conducting a census (all the in-patients in the hospital) on that day. The important indicators are the following:

8. Number of in-patients (July 1of the year)
9. Age distribution
10. Sex distribution
11. Diagnostic distribution
12. Mode of admission status (this may be voluntary, certified, observation, or criminal records)
13. Duration of stay

5.6.4   DISCHARGED CASES (YEAR)

The important indicators are the following:

14. Number of discharged cases (year)
15. Result of treatment
16. Hospital death rate

$$\text{Hospital death rate} = \frac{\text{Number of deaths during the year in the hospital} \times 1000}{\text{Number of in-patients on July 1 of the year}}$$

The result of treatment may be classified as recovered, improved, slightly improved, not improved, and expired.

5.6.5   MAN-POWER INDICATORS (JULY 1 OF THE YEAR)

The important indicators are the following:

17. Number of psychiatrists (July 1 of the year)
18. In-patients per psychiatrist

$$\text{In-patients per psychiatrist} = \frac{\text{Number of in-patients on July 1 of the year}}{\text{Number of psychiatrists on July 1 of the year}}$$

5.6.6   EXPENDITURE PATTERN INDICATORS (FINANCIAL YEAR)

The important indicators are the following:

19. Total expenditure on service (financial year)
20. Unit cost (cost per day per patient)

$$\text{Unit cost} = \frac{\text{Total expenditure on service during the financial year}}{\text{Hospital days of the financial year}}$$

The hospital days of the year are the sum of the daily census figures of all the 365 (or 366) days of the year.

5.7   SERVICE INDICATORS OF GOVERNMENT MENTAL HOSPITALS IN INDIA

There are 36 government mental hospitals in India.

5.7.1   OUT-PATIENT SERVICE INDICATORS

Out-patient services indicators of government mental hospitals are given in Table 5.6

TABLE 5.6   Out-patient services indicators of government mental hospitals

Out-patient service indicators

1. Number of new Registrations (2002): Ranged from 27 to 9215 at individual hospitals		
2. Age (%):	Below 17	15.4
	17–60	81.0
	Above 60	3.6
3. Sex (%)	Male (%):	67.1
	Female (%):	32.9
4. Diagnosis (%):		
	Organic psychoses	2.5
	Substance use disorders	6.4
	Schizophrenia	49.5

TABLE 5.6   *(Continued)*

Mania	6.6
Bipolar affective disorders	12.5
Endogenous depression	7.5
Phobic neuroses	0.4
Anxiety neuroses	1.9
Obsessive compulsive neuroses:	0.7
Neurotic depression	2.8
Dissociative disorders	0.5
Somatoform disorders	0.4
Behavioral disorders	0.3
Personality disorders	0.2
Mental retardation	4.4
Developmental disorders	0.1
Behr./emotional disorders	0.3
Epilepsy	3.0
5. Rate of follow-up attendance	4.5

5.7.2   IN-PATIENT SERVICE INDICATORS

In-patient services indicators of government mental hospitals are given in Table 5.7

TABLE 5.7   In-patient services indicators of government mental hospitals

Admitted patients:

6. Number of admitted patients: Ranged from 12 to 5149 at individual hospitals

7. Rate of admission (%):   38.0

In-patients service indicators:

8. Number of in-patients: Ranged from 19 to 2411 at individual hospitals

9. Age (%):	Below 17	1.8
	17–60	88.7
	Above 60	9.5

10. Sex: (%):	Male	53.0
	Female	47.0
11. Diagnosis (schizophrenia %):		62.1
12. Mode of admission status (%):		
	Voluntary	56.3
	Certified	37.2
	Observation	4.0
	Criminal	2.5
13. Duration of staying: (%)		
	Below 2 years	52.4
	2–5 years	17.6
	5–15 years	18.1
	Above 15 years	11.9

Discharged cases:

14. Number of discharged cases (2012): Ranging from 10 to 5257at individual hospitals

15. Result of treatment (%):

	Recovered	17.2
	Improved	50.8
	Slightly improved	29.1
	Not improved	2.0
	Expired	0.9
16. Hospital Death Rate:		33.0

5.8   SERVICE INDICATORS OF GENERAL HOSPITAL PSYCHIATRIC UNITS

5.8.1   OUT-PATIENT SERVICE INDICATORS

Out-patient service indicators of general hospital psychiatric units are given in Table 5.8

TABLE 5.8 Out-patient service indicators of general hospital psychiatric units

Out-patient service indicators:

1. Number of new registrations: Ranged from 59 to 2514 at individual hospitals

2. Age (%):	Below 17	23.8
	17–60	70.2
	Above 60	6.0
3. Sex (%)	Male (%):	41.0
	Female (%):	59.0
4. Diagnosis (%):		
	Organic psychoses	4.9
	Substance use disorders	10.7
	Schizophrenia	20.3
	Mania	2.5
	Bipolar affective disorders	4.5
	Endogenous depression	20.8
	Phobic neuroses	1.6
	Anxiety neuroses	7.1
	Obsessive compulsive neuroses:	1.9
	Neurotic depression	4.6
	Dissociative disorders	4.0
	Somatoform disorders	4.5
	Behavioral disorders	2.5
	Personality disorders	0.8
	Mental retardation	5.1
	Developmental disorders	0.7
	Behr./emotional disorders	1.6
	Epilepsy	1.9
5. Rate of follow-up attendance		2.1

5.9   OPTIMIZATION OF SERVICE INDICATORS

The reduction in the heterogeneity of important service indicators among the government mental hospitals will optimize the services rendered by these hospitals in any country. The optimization process has both clinical and economic implications.

5.9.1   REDDY'S METHOD

The optimum service indicators of a government mental hospital may be determined as follows:
1. Minimum number of registrations = Number of in-patients x Rate of registrations of all the hospitals in the country.
   where rate of registration = Number of registrations during the year / Number of in-patients as on first July of the year
2. Total follow-up attendences = Number of new registrations x Rate of follow-up attendance of all the hospitals
3. Number of admissions = Number of registrations x Rate of admissions of all the hospitals
4. Maximum number of chronic patients = Number of in-patients x Propotion of chronic patients of all the hospitals

Example : In India for 400 in-patients (Bed strength) as on first July of the year, the optimum indicators are calculated as follows.

Minimum number of new registrations = $400 \times 12 = 4800$
Total follow-up attendance = $4800 \times 4.5 = 21600$
Number of admissions = $4800 \times 0.38 = 1440$
Maximum number of chronic patients = $400 \times 0.476 = 190$

KEYWORDS

- **Demography**
- **Mental morbidity**
- **Prevalence rate**
- **Service indicators**

CHAPTER 6

PROBABILITY AND PROBABILITY DISTRIBUTIONS

CONTENTS

6.1   PROBABILITY SCALE

The probability is the degree of confidence in the occurrence of events. It is the measurement of events. This measure being a number lies between 0 and 1. Thus,

$P = 0$ implies that the occurrence of the event is impossible

$P = 1$ implies that the occurrence of the event is certain

$P = 0.5$ implies that 50 percent chance for the event to occur.

6.1.1   DEFINITIONS OF PROBABILITY

6.1.1.1   THEORETICAL PROBABILITY

The theoretical (mathematical, classical, a priori) probability of occurrence of an event is given by

$$P(E) = \frac{\text{Number of favourable cases}}{\text{Number of possible cases}}$$

Example: In tossing a coin, there are two possible cases: occurrence of head and occurrence of tail. Let us suppose that the occurrence of head is favourable to us. Then,

$P(\text{head}) = \dfrac{1}{2} = 0.5$ or 50%

6.1.1.2   PRACTICAL PROBABILITY

The practical (statistical, empirical, frequency, a posteriori) probability is given by

$$P(E) = \frac{\text{Number of times the event has occured}}{\text{Total number of trials}}$$

Example: There are 24 males in a total of 40 psychiatric registrations at NIMHANS hospital (data in Appendix I).Then, the probability that a registered patient happens to be a male is obtained by

$$P(\text{male}) = \frac{24}{40} = 0.60 \text{ or } 60\%$$

6.1.2   LAWS OF PROBABILITY

6.1.2.1   ADDITION LAW

If two events A and B are mutually exclusive, then the probability of the event "A or B" is given by the sum of their probabilities. That is,

$$P(A \text{ or } B) = P(A) + P(B)$$

Example: It is found that 20 percent of psychiatric registrations at NIMHANS hospital are children (aged below 17 years) and that 10 percent of the registrations are aged (above 60 years). Then, the probability that a registered patient happens to be either a child or aged is obtained as follows:

$$P(\text{child or aged}) = P(\text{child}) + P(\text{aged})$$
$$= 0.20 + 0.10 = 0.30 \text{ or } 30\%$$

6.1.2.2   MULTIPLICATION LAW

If two events A and B are mutually independent, then the probability of the event "A and B" is given by the product of their probabilities. That is,

$$P(A \text{ and } B) = P(A) \times P(B)$$

Example: Let us consider two consecutively registered psychiatric patients at NIMHANS registration counter. The probability that both of them happen to be males is obtained (data in Appendix I) as

$$P(\text{male and male}) = 0.6 \times 0.6 = 0.36 \text{ or } 36\%$$

6.1.2.3   COMPLEMENTARY PROBABILITY

If A is an event, not-A is called its complementary event, and it is denoted by A'. Its probability called complementary probability is given by

$$P(A') = 1 - P(A)$$

Example: The probability that a registered patient at NIMHANS hospital happens to be a female is given by

$$P(\text{female}) = 1 - P(\text{male}) = 1 - 0.60 = 0.40 \text{ or } 40\%$$

6.1.2.4 CONDITIONAL PROBABILITY

If the event A can occur only when it is known that B has occurred, then the occurrence of A is conditional to the occurrence of B. The conditional probability of A given that B has already occurred is obtained by

$$P(A/B) = \frac{P(AB)}{P(B)}$$

where P(AB) is the probability of occurrence of the event.

Example: It is found that 0.4 percent ($P = 0.004$) of psychiatric registrations at NIMHANS hospital have puerperal psychosis and that 40 percent ($P = 0.4$) of the registered patients are females. Then, the probability that a registered patient has puerperal psychosis given that the patient is a female is obtained by

$$P(\text{puerperal psychosis/female}) = \frac{0.004}{0.4} = 0.01 \text{ or } 1\%$$

6.1.3 BAYES THEOREM

In general, the psychiatrist knows the probability of occurrence of a particular symptom in a patient with a particular psychiatric disorder (d). However, it is important to know the probability of occurrence of a particular psychiatric disorder in a patient who has a particular symptom. A theorem attributed to Thomas Bayes may be used to provide the latter probability from the former probability.

6.1.3.1 FORMULA

It is given by

$$P(d/s) = \frac{P(d) \times P(\frac{s}{d})}{P(d) \times P\left(\frac{s}{d}\right) + P(d') \times P(\frac{s}{d'})}$$

Example: It is found that 28 percent of children registered at CGC of NIMHAMS hospital have conduct disorder. Consider the two events that a child has conduct disorder and that the child has non-conduct disorder. It is further known that 63 percent of the conduct disorder children and 17 percent of the non-conduct disorders children of the clinic have truancy at home/school. Then, the probability that a registered child has conduct disorder knowing that the child has truancy is given by

$$P(\text{conduct disorder/truancy}) = \frac{0.28 \times 0.63}{(0.28 \times 0.63) + (0.72 \times 0.17)} = \frac{0.1764}{0.2988} = 0.59 \text{ or } 59\%$$

6.1.4 EVALUATION OF SCREENING TESTS

6.1.4.1 SENSITIVITY AND SPECIFICITY

The sensitivity of screening test is the ability of the test to detect positive cases. That is, the sensitivity is the probability that the screening test indicates a diseased case as positive. The specificity of screening test is the ability of the test to detect negative cases. That is, the specificity is the probability that the screening test indicates a nondiseased case as negative.

A 2 × 2 screening test table

Screening test	Disease	Non-disease
Positive	Truc positive (TP)	False positive (FP)
Negative	False negative (FN)	True negative (TN)
Total	(D)	(ND)

Now,

Sensitivity of the test $= \dfrac{\text{TP}}{\text{(D)}}$

Specificity of the test $= \dfrac{\text{TN}}{\text{(ND)}}$

6.1.5 DEALING WITH CONFIDENTIAL INFORMATION

The estimation of parameters in case of sensitive (confidential) information is unduly affected by the presence of high rate of false answers. This requires an indirect way of obtaining data for a reliable estimate of parameters.

Example: Let us suppose that we are interested in estimating the probability of premarital sex among married women at a psychiatric clinic.

A: Select a random number from 1 to 10. If it is greater than 3, then answer to question B. Otherwise, answer to question C.

B: Have you had premarital sex?

C: Toss a coin. Is it head?

Let us suppose that there are 25 'yes' responses in a total of 100 trials. Then,

$$\frac{25}{100} = P(B \text{ and Yes}) + P(C \text{ and Yes})$$

$$= 0.7\,P + 0.3 \times 0.5$$
$$= 0.7\,P + 0.15$$
$$0.7\,P = 0.25 - 0.15 = 0.10$$

$$P = \frac{0.10}{0.70} = 0.143 \text{ or } 14.3\%$$

6.2   PROBABILITY DISTRIBUTIONS

The statistical inferences are drawn by considering sampling distributions and calculating probabilities. The sampling distributions differ according to the type of the characteristic studied, the nature of the population, and the size of the sample. For each type of situation, a sampling distribution may be formed by using a mathematical modal called theoretical distribution. In several situations, the observed sampling distributions are very close approximation of the theoretical distributions. The mathematical models have been developed, and the required probabilities were calculated and made available by means of tables for certain types of distributions.

6.2.1   BINOMIAL DISTRIBUTION

Sometimes, the psychiatrists are interested to know the proportion of individuals in population possess a particular character such as the number of psychiatric patients in a family of two members. An estimate of this proportion is calculated based on a suitably drawn sample and the corresponding sampling distribution. In this type of problem, the sampling distribution is given by a theoretical frequency distribution known as binominal distribution. It is given by

$$P(x) = n \, C_x \, p^x \, q^{n-x}$$

where

n is the sample size

x is the number of individuals who possess the event

p is the probability of occurrence of the event

$$q = 1-p$$

The nC_x denotes the number of combinations in a set of n objects taken x at a time. It is given by

$$nC_x = \frac{n!}{(n-x)!x!}$$

where $n! = 1 \times 2 \times \ldots \times n$

Example: It is found that the probability of a male registered patient at NIMHANS hospital is 0.60. A sample of two patients at the registration counter can be any one of three types: having no male patient, one male patient, or two male patients. The probabilities of these can be obtained by using binominal probability distribution formula as shown below:

$P(O) = 2Co(0.6)^0(0.4)^2 = 1 \times 1 \times 0.16 = 0.16$

$P(1) = 2C_1(0.6)^1(0.4)^1 = 2 \times 0.6 \times 0.4 = 0.48$

$P(2) = 2C_2(0.6)^2(0.4)^0 = 1 \times 0.36 \times 1 = 0.36$

6.2.2 POISSON DISTRIBUTION

There are situations in which the number of times an event occurs can be counted, but the number of times the event did not occur cannot be counted. For example, the number of follow-ups made by a psychiatric patient may be counted, but this is not possible when the number of follow-ups is not made. The probabilities of observing no follow-up, one follow-up, two follow-ups, and so on, in a given sample of such patients can theoretically be found out by the using Poisson distribution. It is given by

$$P(x) = \frac{e^{-m}m^x}{x!}$$

where x is the number of times the event occurred

m is the mean of the distribution

6.2.3   NORMAL DISTRIBUTION

In many situations, the characteristics (variables) to be studied are continuously measured such as intelligence quotient or IQ, body temperature, etc. For such variables, many populations, and also their sampling distributions, are very close to a pattern of frequency distribution known as normal distribution. The normal distribution is denoted by $N(\bar{x}, \sigma^2)$. The mathematical function that generates the probabilities is given in the literature. An ideal normal distribution curve is as shown in Figure 6.1

FIGURE 6.1   Probability of standard normal values of an observation falling ± 1.96.

An ideal normal distribution curve is symmetrical. About 95 percent of the observations lie within 1.96 standard error from either side of the mean, and about 99 percent of the observations lie within 2.58 standard error from either side of the mean.

6.2.3.1   CENTRAL LIMIT THEOREM

The central limit theorem states that the statistics of all distributions follow normal distribution provided the sample size is sufficiently large. Many variables encountered in psychiatric research have approximate normal distribution. If the distribution is approximately normal, no essential details are lost by considering it to be normal. The mean and standard deviation describe the normal distribution completely.

6.2.4 STANDARD ERRORS OF STATISTICS

The sampling distribution of the statistics calculated from samples taken from the parent normal distribution is known. If a series of samples of fixed size is taken, say n from the population, then the sample means cluster closely around the population mean. The standard deviation of statistic is known as standard error (SE). The SE decreases with an increase in the sample size.

6.2.4.1 STANDARD ERROR OF SAMPLE MEAN

It is given by

$$SE(\overline{x}) = \frac{s}{\sqrt{n}}$$

Example: The SE of the mean of the marks scored by five students (7, 4, 1, 3, and 5) is calculated as follows:

$$SE(\overline{x}) = \frac{\sqrt{5}}{\sqrt{5}} = 1$$

6.2.4.2 STANDARD ERROR OF SAMPLE PROPORTION

It is given by

$$SE(p) = \sqrt{\frac{pq}{n}}$$

Example: The standard error of the proportion of males ($p = 0.6$) in total of 40 registered patients (data in Appendix I) is calculated as follows:

$$SE(p) = \sqrt{\frac{(0.6 \times 0.4)}{40}} = \sqrt{0.006} = 0.077$$

6.2.5 DERIVED DISTRIBUTIONS

Several probability distributions have been developed from the parent normal distribution.

6.2.5.1 STANDARDIZED VALUES

If x is a normal variate, then the standard normal variate or relative normal variate (denoted by Z) is defined as follows:

$$Z = \frac{(x - \bar{x})}{S}$$

The mean of the standard normal values in a dataset is 0 and the standard deviation is 1. The standardized distribution is denoted by $N(0,1)$. The proportions under the entire standard normal curve that lies between 0 and a positive value of Z are presented in probability distribution tables (Appendix III). The proportion of areas between zero and a negative value of Z are obtained by symmetry.

Example: The standardized marks scored by the five students (7, 4, 1, 3, and 5) are computed as shown in the following table.

Student	x	$(x - \bar{x})$	Z
1	7	3	1.5
2	4	0	0
3	1	−3	−1.5
4	3	−1	−0.5
5	5	1	0.5
Mean	4	0	0

6.1.5.2 χ^2(chi-square) DISTRIBUTION

It is the sum of squares of n independent standard normal variates. Given a fixed total in a contingency table, the number of independent cells that can be varied freely will be the number of degrees of freedom (df).

6.1.5.3 t-DISTRIBUTION

It is the ratio of a standard normal variate to the square root of the χ^2 divided by their respective degrees of freedom. The size of the sample minus the number of parameters estimated is called the degree of freedom. Thus, it is the number of independent members in the sample.

6.1.5.4 F-DISTRIBUTION

It is the ratio of two independent χ^2 divided by their respective degree of freedom. Thus, the distribution has two independent degrees of freedom: one attached to the numerator and the other attached to the denominator.

KEYWORDS

- **Bayes theorem**
- **Sampling distribution**
- **Screening tests**
- **Standard error**

SAMPLING THEORY AND METHODS

CONTENTS

7.1   THEORY OF SAMPLING

7.1.1   RANDOM SAMPLING

Generally, we are interested in representative sample to draw valid conclusions on the population. Such representation can be assured only through random sampling. In random sampling, every unit in the population has a known probability of being included in the sample. The sample is drawn by some method of random selection consistent with these probabilities, and we take into account of these probabilities while estimating the parameters. In random sampling, it is possible to study the bias and error attached to the estimates from different sampling techniques. In this way, much has been reported about the scope, advantages, and limitations of each sampling technique so as to choose the one that suits our sampling job reasonably well.

7.1.2   NON-RANDOM SAMPLING

Non-random sampling techniques such as convenient sampling, judgment sampling, and quota sampling do not assure fair representation of the population, and hence they must be based on certain specific purposes.

7.1.3   SAMPLING ERROR

In random sampling, there are sampling errors due to sample enumeration instead of complete enumeration (census enumeration). That is, the sampling errors are the errors of estimates that arise solely from the sampling variation that is present whenever a sample of n units (sample) is measured instead of the complete population of N units (population size). The sampling errors may be reduced by selecting suitable random sampling method, fixing optimum sampling size, and eliminating sample bias.

7.1.4   SAMPLING BIAS

The sampling bias is nothing but consistent errors that arise due to the sample selection. It may be due to wrong demarcation of the sample from the population, measuring the succeeding or proceeding units in the list, and the errors of estimation. Sampling bias means that the data collected may not represent one group.

7.2   RANDOM SAMPLING METHODS

Several random sampling methods are available depending on the objectives of the study, the size and nature of the population, required precision of the estimates, sanctioned budget, and the availability of the sampling frame. A sampling frame is a list of all the units in the population listed alphabetically or chronologically and numbered serially.

7.2.1   SIMPLE RANDOM SAMPLING

This is the simplest of all the random sampling methods. In simple random sampling, each unit in the population has the same chance of being included in the sample at the first draw or at each subsequent draws. The sampling may be carried out by using random number tables or by lottery system of drawing. This sampling method is appropriate when the population size is small, sampling units are homogeneous, and the frame is readily available as in the case of clinical trials.

7.2.1.1   ESTIMATE

An unbiased estimate of the population mean is given by

$$\overline{y}_{SRS} = \frac{1}{n}\sum y_i$$

where n is the sample size
y_i is the observed value of the ith observation
Random numbers: A list of random numbers is given below:

6	8	2	3	6	0	3	9	2	8	9	1	2	3	9	3	8	9	6	4	1	5	3
1	3	2	3	6	5	4	5	2	3	7	9	1	0	5	3	2	7	2	1	5	1	1
0	5	2	4	3	8	6	7	1	3	2	9	2	3	2	5	2	7	9	3	6	5	7
9	0	5	1	0	9	8	9	6	8	0	3	7	9	2	0	5	1	5	1	6	9	4

7.2.2 SYSTEMATIC SAMPLING

The systematic sampling is operationally more convenient than simple random sampling and at the same time ensures equal probability to each unit in the population of being inclusion in the sample. Let $k = N/n$, where N is the population size. k is taken as the nearest integer to N/n. Select a random number from 1 to k, say r. Then, the rth, $(r + k)$th, $\{r + (n - 1)k\}$ th units are selected for the sample. The k is known as sampling interval that is the reciprocal of the sampling fraction, and the random number r is known as random start. This sampling procedure is not valid when there is a periodicity of a particular event under study in the population.

7.2.2.1   ESTIMATE

An unbiased estimate of the population mean is given by

$$\bar{y}_{SYS} = \frac{1}{n}\sum y_i$$

7.2.3   STRATIFIED SAMPLING

Stratified sampling may be preferred to increase the precision of the estimate by reducing the heterogeneity of the population. In stratified sampling, the population of N units is divided into L Sub-populations of N_1, N_2, ... N_L units that are internally homogeneous. These sub-populations are not overlapping, and together they comprise the whole population. The classes into which the population is divided are called strata. Then, each stratum will be sub-sampled, and a definite number of units are taken from each stratum as in the case of simple random sampling. The partial samples of the different strata may be used to estimate the means of several strata from which the overall estimate of the population mean may be obtained.

7.2.3.1 ESTIMATE

An unbiased estimate of the population mean is given by

$$\bar{y}_{ST} = \sum W_h \bar{y}_h$$

where

$$W_h = \frac{N_h}{N}$$

$$\bar{y}_h = \frac{1}{n_h} \sum y_{hi}$$

The n_h is the sample size for the h^{st} stratum. Various allocation models are available in fixing the sample size for each stratum, such as proportional allocation model, etc.

7.2.4 CLUSTER SAMPLING

It consists in forming suitable clusters of units and surveying all the units in a sample of selected cluster. By cluster sampling, it means sampling of clusters of units formed by grouping neighboring units or units that can be surveyed together. For example, while surveying a random sample of schools in a particular city to determine scholastic backwardness of first-grade students in the city. The units within the clusters should be as heterogeneous as possible. Let us deal with the case in which all the clusters are of equal size. Suppose a finite population of NM units is divided into L clusters of size M in each cluster. A sample of n clusters is selected from N clusters using simple random sampling without replacement.

7.2.4.1   ESTIMATE

An unbiased estimate of the population mean is given by

$$\bar{y}_c = \frac{1}{n}\sum \bar{y}_i$$

where $\bar{y}_i = \dfrac{1}{M}\sum y_{ij}$

7.2.5   AREA SAMPLING

Area sampling is close to cluster sampling, which is more suitable for mental morbidity surveys. Under area sampling, we first divide the total area into a number of smaller non-overlapping areas called geographical clusters, then a number of these clusters are randomly selected, and all the units in the selected clusters are included in that sample.

7.3   RANDOM SAMPLING METHODS IN MENTAL MORBIDITY SURVEYS

The mental morbidity surveys in India adapted the following schemes of selection of study areas/sampling procedures depending on the nature of the population (general or specific).

7.3.1   RURAL SECTORS

For rural sectors, the schemes of selection of study areas/sampling procedures are the following:
- A part of the village
- A single village
- Villages in two wards of a *panchayat*
- All families of three communities in clusters of small villages
- A random sample of families from four villages
- A random sample of 50 percent of families in 11 villages of a block

7.3.2   URBAN SECTORS

For urban sectors, the schemes of selection of study areas/sampling procedures are the following:
- A random sample of families from urban health center
- A slum locality in a metropolitan city

7.3.3   SEMI-URBAN SECTORS

For semi-urban sectors, the schemes of selection of study areas/sampling procedures are as follows:
- A sample of families of officers staying in their official quarters in a particular area of a city
- A sample of families of a tribal community migrated to an urban area

KEYWORDS

- **Sampling bias**
- **Sampling methods**

CHAPTER 8

BASIC ELEMENTS OF STATISTICAL INFERENCE

CONTENTS

8.1   BASIC ELEMENTS OF ESTIMATION OF PARAMETERS

An estimator is a function of sample values, whereas an estimate is a numerical value of the estimator. An estimate may be a single statistic (such as the sample mean for a population mean, sample proportion for a population proportion, etc.), which is called point estimates or a range with attached probabilities called interval estimates or confidence intervals.

8.1.1   POINT ESTIMATES

The criteria for selecting a suitable estimator for a purpose have to be described.

8.1.1.1 CONSISTENCY, EFFICIENCY, AND SUFFICIENCY

A consistent estimator gets increasingly better as the sample size increases. For example, the sample mean and the median are consistent estimators of their respective parameters. An efficient estimator is one for which the standard error is small. In many situations, the sample mean tends to be more efficient estimator than the sample median, although there are situations for which the reverse is also true. A sufficient estimator makes use of all the potentially useful information in the data. Thus, the sample mean is a sufficient estimator, but not the sample median.

8.1.1.2   RESISTANCE

A resistant estimator is not affected too much by the presence of extreme values or the outliers in the data. For example, the sample median is a resistant estimator, but not the sample mean. We should pay particular attention to resistant estimator in psychiatric research since gross errors or outliers occur frequently in practice.

8.1.1.3   UNBIASED

The expected value of an unbiased estimator is equal to the parameter value. The expected value of a random variate is given by

$$E(x) = \sum x_i p_i$$

where x_1 are the sampling points

p_1 are the attached probabilities of the sampling points

Example: The expected value when a die is rolled is calculated as follows:

$$E \text{ (die)} = (1 + 2 + 3 + 4 + 5 + 6)/6 = 21/6 = 3.5$$

The sample mean $(\overline{x})$ is an unbiased estimator of the population mean (μ). An unbiased estimator of standard deviation of sample is given by

$$s = \sqrt{\frac{1}{(n-1)}\sum(x-\overline{x})^2}$$

Example: The unbiased standard deviation for five values (7, 4, 1, 3, and 5) is calculated as follows:

$$s = \sqrt{\frac{20}{4}} = \sqrt{5} = 2.236$$

Whereas the biased estimator for the same data has been calculated as follows:

$$S = \sqrt{\frac{20}{5}} = \sqrt{4} = 2.0$$

8.1.2   INTERVAL ESTIMATES

The estimation of confidence interval (CI) is important since the investigator can never estimate the exact values of the parameter with certainty. The procedure is to obtain a point estimate and then set up certain limits on both sides of the estimate on the basis of the sampling distribution of the statistics used. Thus, the CI helps in locating the parameter values. The sample mean $(\overline{x})$ is the best point estimator for population mean (μ).

8.1.2.1 CI FOR MEAN

When the sample size is large (more than 30), the 95 percent CI for estimating population mean is given by

$$\bar{x} \pm 1.96 \times SE\left(\bar{x}\right)$$

That is,

$$\bar{x} \pm 1.96 \times \frac{s}{\sqrt{n}}$$

when the sample size is small, the 95 percent CI is given by

$$\bar{x} \pm t \times SE\left(\bar{x}\right)$$

Example: The 95 percent CI for the marks scored by the five students(7, 4, 1, 3, and 5) is worked out as follows:

$$4 \pm 2.78 \times 1, \text{ that is } 1.22 \text{ to } 6.78$$

where the table value of $t\,(4) = 2.78$, at 5 percent level of significance.

8.1.2.2 CI FOR PROPORTION

The sample proportion (p) is the best estimator of the population proportion (P). When the sample size is large, the 95 percent CI for estimating population proportion is given by

$$p \pm 1.96 \times SE\,(p)$$

That is,

$$p \pm 1.96 \times \sqrt{\frac{pq}{n}}$$

Example: The 95 percent CI for population proportion of male patients at NIMHANS registration (data in Appendix I) is worked out as follows:

$$0.6 \pm 1.96 \times 0.077$$

$$0.6 \pm 0.15, \text{ that is, } 0.45 \text{ to } 0.75$$

8.1.3   DETERMINATION OF SAMPLE SIZE

The sampling variance decreases with increase in the sample size; but at the same time, the cost of the survey also increases. Hence, in practice, the optimum sample size that decreases the sampling error for a reasonable cost has to be determined. The general relationship between the sample size and sampling error is as shown in the Figure 8.1.

FIGURE 8.1   General relationship between sample size and sampling error.

8.1.3.1   SAMPLE SIZE FOR ESTIMATING POPULATION MEAN

In case of estimating a population mean, the optimum sample size is determined by

$$n = \frac{Z_\alpha^2 S^2}{d^2}$$

where Z_α is fixed at 1.96 for 5 percent level of significance

S^2 is the estimate of the variance from a pilot study

d is the allowable error (difference from the true value) due to sampling defects that can be tolerated. It is usually fixed at 10 percent of the available estimate from the pilot study.

Example: Let us support that the marks scored by a randomly selected five students in a test are 7, 4, 1, 3, and 5. Then, the sample size required for estimating the population mean is determined as follows:

$$n = \frac{1.96^2 \times 5}{(4 \times 0.1)^2} = \frac{3.841 \times 5}{0.16} = \frac{19.205}{0.16} = 120$$

8.1.3.2   SAMPLE SIZE FOR ESTIMATING POPULATION PROPORTION

In case of estimating a population proportion, the optimum sample size is determined as follows:

$$n = \frac{Z_\alpha^2 pq}{d^2}$$

where p is the available estimate of the proportion

Example: The sample size required for estimating the proportion of males at NIMHANS psychiatric registrations (data in Appendix I) is given by

$$n = \frac{1.96^2 \times 0.6 \times 0.4}{(0.6 \times 0.1)^2} = \frac{3.841 \times 0.24}{0.0036} = 256, \text{ or approximately } 260$$

8.2   BASIC ELEMENTS OF TESTS OF SIGNIFICANCE

A researcher involves in making hypothesis about population and checking the plausibility of the hypothesis using sample data. The sampling variation is considered in this process.

8.2.1   NULL AND ALTERNATE HYPOTHESES

The assumption of no difference between populations or no association between factors in the population is known as null hypothesis and is denoted by H_0. When the null hypothesis is rejected, the other hypothesis $(H_1, H_2, …)$ known as alternate hypothesis has to be accepted.

8.2.2   STATISTICAL SIGNIFICANCE

This means that the difference between the observed score from the sample and the score based on the hypothesis is not due to chance, defying the null hypothesis. On the contrary, the statistic is not significant means that the difference is obtained by chance.

8.2.3   TYPE I AND TYPE II ERRORS

Type I error rejects the null hypothesis when it is actually true, whereas type II error accepts the null hypothesis when it is actually false. A table showing the type I error and type II error is as given below:

	H_0 is true	H_0 is false
Action taken: Reject	Type I error	-
Accept	-	Type II error

8.2.4   LEVEL OF SIGNIFICANCE AND POWER OF THE TEST

The probability of committing type I error is known as the level of significance. That is,

$$\text{Level of significance} = P \text{ (type I error)}$$

It is usually fixed at 5 percent ($P = 0.05$).The power of the test is the probability of rejecting the false null hypothesis. Thus, the power of the test is given by

$$\text{Power of the test} = 1 - P \text{ (type II error)}$$

Thus, the power of the test is the probability of rejecting the false null hypothesis. Experience suggests that in practice the power of the test is set at a maximum of 80 percent.

8.2.5   TWO-TAILED AND ONE-TAILED TESTS

In test of significances when we want to determine, for example, whether the mean age of onset of schizophrenia is different from that of bipolar affective disorders, and does not specify higher or lower, the P-values include both sides of extreme result, and the test is called two-tailed test. In case of 5 percent level of significance, the P-values will be 2.5 percent at each end. Therefore, the result is compared with the table value at the probability level of 0.05. The difference is being tested for significance, but the direction is not specified. When we want to test, for example, whether the mean of schizophrenia is less than that of bipolar affective disorders, the results will be at one end of the tail of the distribution, and the test is called one-tailed test.

8.2.6   TEST STATISTIC

In statistical hypothesis testing, a hypothesis test is typically specified in terms of test statistic that is a function of the sample. It is considered as a numerical summary of a set of data that reduces the data to one or a small number of values that can be used to perform a hypothesis test.

8.2.7   STEPS INVOLVED IN STATISTICAL TESTS OF SIGNIFICANCE

There are various types of problems for which the test of significance are used for drawing conclusions. Different types of problem require different tests, but the basis and the steps involved in the procedures are one and the same.

1. Stating the null hypothesis and the alternate hypotheses.
2. Formulate statistic and calculate its standard error. That is, calculate the critical ratio and determine its distribution.
3. Compare the observed value of the critical ratio with that of the table value at 5 and 1 percent level of significance. If the calculated value is less than the table value, then accept the null hypothesis. If the calculated value is more than the table value, then reject the null hypothesis and accept the alternate hypothesis.

KEYWORDS

- **Confidence interval**
- **Point estimates**
- **Resistant estimator**
- **Statistical tests**

CHAPTER 9

PARAMETRIC TESTS OF SIGNIFICANCE

CONTENTS

9.1 ONE-SAMPLE PARAMETRIC TESTS

9.1.1 ONE-SAMPLE *t*-TEST

9.1.1.1 HYPOTHESES

The one-sample *t*-test is applied to test for a population mean. It compares the mean score of a sample ($\overline{x}$) to an unknown value (μ_0). The unknown value is a population mean. That is,

H_0: $\mu = \mu_0$ against H_1: $\mu \neq \mu_0$

9.1.1.2 TEST STATISTIC

It is given by

$$t = \frac{|\overline{x} - \mu_0|}{s / \sqrt{n}} \text{ with df} = (n{-}1)$$

9.1.1.3 SAMPLE SIZE

The optimum sample size is determined by

$$n = \frac{\left(Z_\alpha + Z_\beta\right)^2 S^2}{\left(\overline{x} - \mu_0\right)^2}$$

where $Z_\alpha = 1.96$ and $Z_\beta = 0.84$

Example: Let us assume that the improvement scores of a group of five patients in a test are given by 7, 4, 1, 3, and 5. We wish to test whether the mean score of the whole class can be considered as 5.0. That is,

$$t = \frac{|4-5|}{\sqrt{5} / \sqrt{5}} = 1.0, \text{ with df} = (5{-}1) = 4$$

where $s = \sqrt{5}$

Since the calculated value is less than the table value of $t(4) = 2.78$ at 5 percent level of significance, we accept the null hypothesis ($P > 0.05$, not significant).

For this data,

$$n = \frac{(1.96 + 0.84\ )^2 \times 5}{(4-5)^2} = 2.8^2 \times 5 = 39.2$$

Thus, the sample size required for this purpose is about 40.

9.1.2 ONE-SAMPLE PROPORTION TEST

9.1.2.1 HYPOTHESES

The one-sample proportion test is applied to test for a population proportion. It compares the sample proportion (p) to a known proportion (P_0). That is,

$$H_0{:}P = P_0 \text{ against } H_1{:}\ P \neq P_0 \text{ (large sample)}$$

9.1.2.2 TEST STATISTIC

This is given by the following relation:

$$Z = \frac{|\, p - P_0 \,|}{\sqrt{P_0 Q_0 / n}}$$

where n is the sample size
  p is the observed sample proportion
  P_0 is the proportion under the null hypothesis

$$Q_0 = 1 - P_0$$

9.1.2.3 SAMPLE SIZE

In testing for a population proportion, the optimum sample size is determined by the following relation:

$$n = \left(\frac{Z_\alpha \sqrt{P_0 Q_0} + Z_\beta \sqrt{pq}}{(p - P_0)} \right)^2$$

Example: A sample of 40 registrations at NIMHANS showed that there are 24 males ($p = 0.6$). We wish to test whether the population proportion can be considered as 0.5. That is,

$H_0: P_0 = 0.50$, against $H_1: P_0 \neq 0.50$.

For this data,

$$Z = \frac{|0.60 - 0.50|}{\sqrt{(0.5 \times 0.5)/40}} = \frac{0.10\sqrt{40}}{0.5} = 1.26$$

Since the calculated value is less that 1.96, we accept the null hypothesis ($P > 0.05$, not significant).

For this data,

$$n = \left(\frac{1.96\sqrt{0.5 \times 0.5} + 0.84\sqrt{0.6 \times 0.4}}{(0.6 - 0.5)} \right) = \left(\frac{0.98 + 0.41}{(0.1)} \right)^2 = 193$$

Thus, the sample size required for the purpose is about 200.

9.2 TWO-INDEPENDENT SAMPLE PARAMETRIC TESTS

9.2.1 INDEPENDENT SAMPLE t-TEST

9.2.1.1 HYPOTHESES

The independent sample *t*-test is applied to test for equality of two population means. It compares the mean scores of two independent samples. That is,

$H_0: \mu_1 = \mu_2$ against $H_1: \mu_1 \neq \mu_2$

9.2.1.2 TEST STATISTIC

It is given by

$$t = \frac{|\bar{x} - \bar{y}|}{\sqrt{\frac{(\sum x^2 - n_1\bar{x}^2) + (\sum y^2 - n_2\bar{y}^2)}{(n_1 + n_2 - 2)} \times \left(\frac{1}{n_1} + \frac{1}{n_2}\right)}}$$

with df $= (n_1 + n_2 - 2)$

9.2.1.3 SAMPLE SIZE

The optimum sample size is given by

$$n = \frac{(Z_\alpha + Z_\beta)^2 S^2}{(\bar{x} - \bar{y})^2}$$

Example: Let us assume that the improvement scores of five randomly selected patients under treatment to be 7, 4, 1, 3, and 5, respectively. The improvement scores of another five randomly selected patients under controls are given by 4, 2, 3, 0, and 6. Here, we wish the test,
H_0: $\mu_1 = \mu_2$ against H_1: $\mu_1 \neq \mu_2$.

$$t = \frac{|4-3|}{\sqrt{\frac{(100 - 5\times 4^2) + (65 - 5\times 3^2)}{(5+5-2)} \times (\frac{1}{5} + \frac{1}{5})}} = \frac{1}{\sqrt{\frac{20+20}{8} \times \frac{2}{5}}} = \frac{1}{\sqrt{2}} = 0.707$$

Since, the calculated value is less than the table value of $t(8) = 2.31$ at 5 percent level of significance, we accept the null hypothesis.
For this purpose,

$$n = \frac{(1.96 + 0.84)^2 \times 5}{(4-3)^2} = 2.8^2 \times 5 = 39.2$$

The sample size required for this test of significance is about 40.

9.2.2 TWO-INDEPENDENT SAMPLE PROPORTION TEST

9.2.2.1 HYPOTHESES

The two-sample proportion test is applied to test for equality of two populations proportions. It compares the proportions of two independent samples. That is,

$H_0: P_1 = P_2$ against $H_1: P_1 \neq P_2$ (large samples)

9.2.2.2   TEST STATISTIC

It is given by

$$Z = \frac{|p_1 - p_2|}{\sqrt{pq\left(\dfrac{1}{n_1} + \dfrac{1}{n_2}\right)}}$$

where $p = \dfrac{n_1 p_1 + n_2 p_2}{(n_1 + n_2)}$ $q = 1 - p$

9.2.2.3   SAMPLE SIZE

In testing for equality of two population proportions, the optimum sample size is determined by

$$n = \left[\frac{Z_\alpha \sqrt{2p_1 q_1} + Z_\beta \sqrt{p_1 q_1 + p_2 q_2}}{(p_1 - p_2)}\right]^2$$

Example: There are 24 males in a random sample of 40 registrations at NIMHANS hospital ($p_1 = 0.60$). There are 28 males in a sample of 40 registrations at KIMHANS (Karnataka Institute of Mental Health and Neroscience, Dharward). That is, ($p_2 = 0.70$). Therefore, we wish to test whether the proportions of male registrations at these two institutes are equal. That is,

$$Z = \frac{|0.6 - 0.7|}{\sqrt{(0.65 \times 0.35)(\dfrac{1}{40} + \dfrac{1}{40})}}$$

$$= \frac{0.1}{\sqrt{0.2275 \times 0.05}} = 0.94$$

Since, the calculated value is less than 1.96, we accept the null hypothesis ($P > 0.05$ not significant).

For this data,

$$n = \left[\frac{1.96\sqrt{2\times0.6\times0.4} + 0.84\sqrt{(0.6\times0.4) + (0.7\times0.3)}}{(0.6-0.7)} \right]^2 = \left[\frac{1.3579 + 0.5635}{-0.1} \right]^2 = 369$$

Thus, the sample size required for the purpose is about 370.

9.3   TWO-RELATED SAMPLE PARAMETRIC TESTS

9.3.1   PAIRED SAMPLE t-TEST

9.3.1.1   HYPOTHESES

It computes the difference between the two sets of scores (scores before giving the treatment and scores after giving the treatment) for each case and tests to see if the average difference is significantly different from 0. That is,

$H_0: \overline{d} = 0$ against $H_1: \overline{d} \neq 0$

where $d = (x - y)$

x are the scores of the persons before giving the treatment

y are the scores of the persons after giving the treatment

9.3.1.2   TEST STATISTIC

It is given by

$$t = \frac{\overline{d}}{s_d / \sqrt{n}} \qquad \text{with df} = (n - 1)$$

where s_d is the unbiased estimate of standard deviation of the differences.

Example: Let us support that the improvement scores of a group of five patients before giving the treatment and the scores after giving the treatment are given below:

Patient	1	2	3	4	5
Before	4	2	3	0	6
After	7	4	1	3	5

The computation table is as given below:

Patient	Before	After	Difference (d)	$(d-\bar{d})$	$(d-\bar{d})^2$
1	4	7	3	2	4
2	2	4	2	1	1
3	3	1	−2	−3	9
4	0	3	3	2	4
5	6	5	−1	−2	4
Total			5		22

$$\bar{d} = \frac{5}{5} = 1.0$$

$$s_{\bar{d}} = \sqrt{\frac{22}{4}} = \sqrt{5.5}$$

$$t = \frac{1}{\sqrt{5.5}/\sqrt{5}} = \frac{1}{\sqrt{1.1}} = 0.953, \text{ with df} = (5-1) = 4$$

Since, the calculated value is less than the table value of $t(4) = 2.78$ at 5 percent level of significance, the null hypothesis is accepted ($P > 0.05$, not significant).

KEYWORDS

- Null hypothesis
- Parametric tests
- *t*-test

CHAPTER 10

EXPERIMENTAL DATA ANALYSIS: ANOVA

CONTENTS

10.1   ONE-WAY ANOVA

10.1.1   LAYOUT

The one-way ANOVA is carried out for data in completely randomized design (CRD). The layout of CRD is as given below:

	Treatment1	Treatment2	-	Treatment k
	x_{11}	x_{21}		x_{k1}
	x_{12}	x_{22}		x_{k2}
	x_{1n_1}	x_{2n_2}		x_{kn_k}
Mean	$\bar{x}_1$	$\bar{x}_2$	-	$\bar{x}_k$

10.1.2   HYPOTHESES

The one-way ANOVA is applied to test for homogeneity of several population means. The null hypothesis states that the population means are homogenous (equal). That is,

$$H_0: \mu_1 = \mu_2 = \ \text{.......} = \mu_k \text{ against } H_1: \mu_i\text{'s are not equal.}$$

10.1.3   TECHNIQUE

The technique consists in estimating two population variances: one is based on between-sample variance called the mean sum of squares between groups or samples (MSS_B) and the other is based on within-sample variance called mean sum of squares within samples (MSS_w). Then, the two estimators are compared with the F-ratio. When the samples come from identical population, these two estimates of the population variances are comparable; any difference observed between them is expected to be within the range of their sampling error. When the populations from which the samples are drawn have different means, the MSS_B is expected to provide a higher value. Symbolically, the technique of ANOVA is given as follows:

$$SS_T = SS_B + SS_W$$

10.1.4 TEST STATISTIC

The test statistic is given by
$$F = \frac{MSS_B}{MSS_W} \text{ with df} = (k - 1, n - k)$$

ANOVA table: It is given by

Sources of variation	df	SS	MSS	F-Ratio
Between treatment	$(k-1)$	SS_B	MSS_B	F
Within treatment	$(n-k)$	SS_w	MSS_w	-
Total	$(n-1)$	SS_T	-	-

where $MSS_B = \dfrac{SS_B}{(k-1)}$

$$MSS_w = \frac{SS_W}{(n-k)}$$

$$SS_B = \sum n_i (\overline{x}_i - \overline{x})^2 = \sum \frac{T_i^2}{n_i} - \frac{T^2}{n}$$

$$SS_w = \sum\sum (X_{ij} - \overline{x}_i)^2 = \sum\sum x_{ij}^2 - \sum \frac{T_i^2}{n_i}$$

Example: Let us suppose that the improvement scores of 15 patients from three different treatments are given below:

Treatment 1	Treatment 2	Treatment 3
4	7	10
2	4	7
3	1	8
0	3	6
6	5	4

For this data, the one-way ANOVA computations are as given below:

Statistics	Treatment 1	Treatment 2	Treatment 3
Sample size	5	5	5
Sum	15	20	35
Mean	3	4	7
Sum of squares	65	100	265

Hence,

$$SS_B = \left(\frac{15^2}{5} + \frac{20^2}{5} + \frac{35^2}{5} \right) - \frac{70^2}{15} = 370 - 326.67 = 43.33$$

$$SS_W = (65 + 100 + 265) - 370 = 430 - 370 = 60$$

Source of variation	df	SS	MSS	F-ratio
Between treatment	2	43.33	21.67	4.33
Within treatment	12	60.00	5.00	-
Total	14	103.33	-	-

Since the calculated value of F is more than the table value of $F(2, 12)$ = 3.89, we reject the null hypothesis at 5 percent level of significance ($P < 0.05$, significant).

10.2 POST-HOC MULTIPLE COMPARISON TESTS: *Scheffé's* METHOD

10.2.1 *HYPOTHESES*

A significance F-test in ANOVA does not mean that every group in the analysis is significantly different from every other group. Sometimes, we are interested in carrying out the test of significance of the difference in pairs of means. The tests applied after finding out that the overall F is significant are called post-hoc tests. Here, the usual Z-values and t-values are cumbersome. The *Scheffé's* method is the commonly used post-hoc test. This method consists in calculating critical value of F (denoted by F_{cv})

to use as a standard against which to compare the differences in pairs of means.

10.2.2   CRITICAL VALUE OF F

It is given by

$$F_{cv} = (k-1)\,F$$
   where k is the number of groups
   F is the value needed to gain significance in the ANOVA

10.2.3   TEST STATISTICS

The test statistics for equality of means of ith group and the jth group in this method is given by

$$F_{(i,j)} = \frac{(\bar{x}_i - \bar{x}_j)^2}{MSS_w\left(\dfrac{1}{n_i} + \dfrac{1}{n_j}\right)}$$

The F is the value needed to gain significance in the ANOVA.

   Example: Let us apply the *Scheffé's* method of post-hoc multiple comparison test to compare pairs of means to the data used to demonstrate the one-way ANOVA.
   Here,

$$F_{cv} = (3-1)\,3.89 = 7.78$$

To compare group 1 and group 2,

$$F_{(1,2)} = \frac{(3-4)^2}{5\left(\dfrac{1}{5}+\dfrac{1}{5}\right)} = \frac{1}{2} = 0.5$$

To compare group 1 and group 3,

$$F_{(1,3)} = \frac{(3-7)^2}{5(\frac{1}{5}+\frac{1}{5})} = \frac{16}{2} = 8.0$$

To compare group 2 and group 3,

$$F_{(2,3)} = \frac{(4-7)^2}{5(\frac{1}{5}+\frac{1}{5})} = \frac{9}{2} = 4.5$$

Since the *Scheffé* $F_{(1,3)}$ is more than F_{cv}, we reject the null hypothesis that the means of first group and the third group are different ($P < 0.05$, significant).

10.3   TWO-WAY ANOVA

10.3.1   LAYOUT

The two-way ANOVA is carried out for data in randomized block design (RBD). The layout of the data collected with this design is as given below:

Blocks	Treatment 1	Treatment 2	-	Treatment k	Mean
1	x_{11}	x_{21}	-	x_{k1}	$\bar{x}.1$
2	x_{12}	x_{22}	-	x_{k2}	$\bar{x}.2$
-	-	-	-	-	-
r	x_{1r}	x_{2r}	-	x_{kr}	$\bar{x}.r$
Mean	$\bar{x}_1.$	$\bar{x}_2.$	-	$\bar{x}_k.$	$\bar{x}$

10.3.2   HYPOTHESES

To test the significance of the means of t treatments effects, and also the significance of the means of r blocks effects. That is,

$H_{01}: t_1 = t_2 = - - = t_k$ against H_{11}: The treatments have different effects

$H_{02}: b_1 = b_2 = - - = b_r$ against H_{12}: The blocks have different effects

10.3.3 TECHNIQUE

The technique consists in dividing the total variance as given below:
$$SS_T = SS_{Tr} + SS_{Bl} + SS_E$$

10.3.4 TEST STATISTICS

They are given by

$$F_{Tr} = \frac{MSS_{Tr}}{MSS_E} \text{ with df} = (k-1), (r-1)(k-1)$$

$$F_{BL} = \frac{MSS_{BL}}{MSS_E} \text{ with df} = (r-1), (r-1)(k-1)$$

Two-Way ANOVA Table

Source of variation	df	SS	MSS	F-ratio
Between treatments	$(k-1)$	SS_{Tr}	MSS_{Tr}	F_{Tr}
Between blocks	$(r-1)$	SS_{Bl}	MSS_{Bl}	F_{Bl}
Error	$(r-1)(k-1)$	SS_E	MSS_E	-
Total	$(rk-1)$	SS_T	-	-

Example: Let us support that the improvement scores of 15 patients from three treatments and five (groups) blocks using RBD is given below:

Blocks	Treatment 1	Treatment 2	Treatment 3	Total	Mean
1	4	7	10	21	7.0
2	2	4	7	13	4.3
3	3	1	8	12	4.0
4	0	3	6	9	3.0
5	6	5	4	15	5.0
Mean	3	4	7	70	4.6

The two-way ANOVA is given by

Source of variation	df	SS	MSS	F-ratio
Between treatment	2	43.33	21.67	5.20
Between blocks	4	26.67	6.67	1.60
Error	8	33.33	4.17	-
Total	14	103.33	-	-

The requisite computations are

$$SS_{Bl} = \frac{1}{3}(21^2 + 13^2 + 12^2 + 9^2 + 15^2) - 326.67$$

$$= \frac{1060}{3} - 326.67 = 353.33 - 326.67 = 26.67$$

Since, the calculated value of F_{Tr} is more than the table value of $F(2,8)$ = 4.46, the null hypothesis is rejected ($P < 0.05$, significant) in cases of treatments.

10.4   2²-FACTORIAL ANOVA

10.4.1   LAYOUT

The layout of the data in 2^2 (or 2×2) factorial experimental design with RBD is given below:

Blocks	1	a	b	ab
1	x_{11}	x_{21}	x_{31}	x_{41}
2	x_{12}	x_{22}	x_{32}	x_{42}
-	-	-	-	-
R	x_{1r}	x_{2r}	x_{3r}	x_{4r}
Total	(1)	(a)	(b)	(ab)

10.4.2   HYPOTHESES

The four treatment combinations can be compared by carry out a 2²-factorial ANOVA.

10.4.3   TECHNIQUE

In 2²-factorial ANOVA, our main objective is to carry out separate test for the main effects A, B, and the interaction AB by splitting the SS_{Tr} with 3 df in three orthogonal components each associated with either with the main effects A and B or the interaction AB, and each with one degree of freedom. That is,

$$SS_{Tr} = SS_A + SS_B + SS_{AB}$$

10.4.4 TEST STATISTICS

The test statistics are given by

$F_A = \frac{MSS_A}{MSS_E}$ with df = 1, $3(r-1)$

$F_B = \frac{MSS_B}{MSS_E}$ with df = 1, $3(r-1)$

$F_{AB} = \frac{MSS_{AB}}{MSS_E}$ with df = 1, $3(r-1)$

where $SS_A = \left(-(1)+(a)-(b)+(ab)\right)^2 / 4r$

$SS_B = \left(-(1)-(a)+(b)+(ab)\right)^2 / 4r$

$SS_{AB} = \left((1)-(a)-(b)+(ab)\right)^2 / 4r$

2^2-Factorial ANOVA Table:

Source of variation	df	SS	MSS	F-ratio
Treatments	3	SS_{Tr}	MSS_{Tr}	F_{Tr}
Main A	1	SS_A	MSS_A	F_A
Main B	1	SS_B	MSS_B	F_B
Interaction AB	1	SS_{AB}	MSS_{AB}	F_{AB}
Blocks	$(r-1)$	SS_{BL}	MSS_{Bl}	F_{Bl}
Errors	$3(r-1)$	SS_E	MSS_E	-
Total	$(4r-1)$	SS_T	-	-

Example: Let us support that there are two different treatments A and B each two levels (not given, given), and hence there are four groups of patients each group consisting of five patients allotted at random to five age groups (2^2-factorial design in RBD). The improvement scores of the 20 patients are given below:

Blocks	Treatments				Mean
	1	a	b	ab	
1	4	7	10	9	7.50
2	2	4	7	12	6.25
3	3	1	8	8	5.00
4	0	3	6	10	4.75
5	6	5	4	6	5.25
Mean	3	4	7	9	5.75

The 2^2-factorial ANOVA table is given below:

Score of variation	df	SS	MSS	F-ratio
Treatment	3	113.75	37.92	7.74
Main A	1	11.25	11.25	2.30
Main B	1	101.25	101.25	20.67
Interaction AB	1	1.25	1.25	0.67
Blocks	4	20.50	5.13	1.05
Errors	12	59.50	4.90	-
Total	19	193.75	-	-

Since the calculated value is more than the table value of $F(3, 12) = 3.49$, the treatments effects are significantly different ($P < 0.05$, significant).

10.5 REPEATED MEASURES ANOVA

10.5.1 LAYOUT

The layout of repeated measures ANOVA design is given by

Subject	Repeat 1	Repeat 2	-	Repeat k
1	x_{11}	x_{21}	-	x_{k1}
2	x_{12}	x_{22}	-	x_{k2}
-	-	-	-	-
n	x_{1n}	x_{2n}	-	x_{kn}

10.5.2 HYPOTHESES

To test homogeneity of means of several repeated measures.

10.5.3 TECHNIQUE

Here, we are interested in refining the experimental design to increase its sensitivity to detect differences in the dependent variable. A major source of experimental error is individual differences that can be controlled by using repeated measures or within-subjects design. By having the same participants perform under every condition, systematic bias attributable to participants in one group being different from the participants in other groups can be eliminated. The assumptions underlying this method are random selection, normality, homogeneity of variance, and sphericity. In this technique,

$$SS_{Rep} = SS_B$$

$$SS_{Res} = SS_W - SS_{Sub}$$

where

$$SS_{Sub} = \sum \frac{T_{.k}^2}{k} - \frac{T^2}{nk}$$

10.5.4 TEST STATISTIC

It is given by

$$F_{Res} = \frac{MSS_{Rep}}{MSS_{Res}}$$

where $SS_{Sub} = \sum \dfrac{T_{.k}^2}{k} - \dfrac{T^2}{nk}$

Repeated Measures ANOVA Table:

Source of variation	df	SS	MSS	F-ratio
Repeated measures	(k-1)	SS_{Rep}	MSS_{Rep}	F_{Rep}
Residuals	(n-1) (k-1)	SS_{Res}	MSS_{Res}	-

Example: Let us suppose that the marks scored by five students in three repeated tests are given below:

Student	Repeat 1	Repeat 2	Repeat 3
1	4	7	10
2	2	4	7
3	3	1	8
4	0	3	6
5	6	5	4

For this data, the repeated measures ANOVA is given below:

Source of variation	df	SS	MSS	F-ratio
Repeated measures	2	43.33	21.67	5.20
Residuals	8	33.33	4.17	-

Since, the calculated value of F is more than the table value of $F(2, 8)$ = 4.46, we reject the null hypothesis ($P < 0.05$, significant)

KEYWORDS

- **ANOVA**
- **Randomized block design**
- ***Scheffé's*** **method**
- **Test statistics**

CHAPTER 11

NON-PARAMETRIC TESTS OF SIGNIFICANCE

CONTENTS

11.1   ONE-SAMPLE NON-PARAMETRIC TESTS

11.1.1   CHI-SQUARE TESTS: 1x K CONTINGENCY TABLE

11.1.1.1   HYPOTHESES

The one-sample chi-square test may be used to test for goodness of fit. It can be applied to decide whether a distribution of a variable in a sample represents or fits a specified population. That is, you can use this test to decide whether your data follows approximate normal distribution, uniform distribution, Poisson distribution, etc.

11.1.1.2   1x K CONTINGENCY TABLE

A table showing bivariate frequency distribution is known as contingency table. The 1×k contingency table has one row and k columns as shown below:

1 x k Contingency Table

Attribute	Category 1	Category2	-	Category k	Total
Observed Frequencies	O_1	O_2	-	O_k	n

11.1.1.3   TEST STATISTIC

It is given by

$$\chi^2 = \sum \frac{(O_i - e_i)^2}{e_i} = \sum \frac{O_i^2}{e_i} - n \text{ with df} = (k-1)$$

where O_i is the observed frequency of the ith category; e_i is the expected frequency of the ith category. They are calculated under the assumption that the null hypothesis is true.

Example: The classification of the 40 registered patients (data in Appendix I) according to the type of locality is given in the following table. We wish to test whether the number of registrations from the three localities can be considered equal.

	rural	semi-urban	urban	Total
Number of patients	16	13	11	40

For this data,

	rural	semi-urban	urban	Total
O_i	16	13	11	40
e_i	13.33	13.33	13.33	40
$(O_i - e_i)$	2.67	−0.33	−2.33	0
$(O_i - e_i)^2$	7.13	0.11	5.43	
$\dfrac{(O_i - e_i)^2}{e_i}$	0.53	0.007	0.398	0.953

Hence,
$\chi^2 = 0.953$, df $= (3-1) = 2$

Since, the calculated value is less than the table value of $\chi^2 = 5.99$ at df $= 2$, we accept the null hypothesis ($P>0.05$, not significant).

11.1.2   CHI-SQUARE TESTS: *R* x *K* CONTINGENCY TABLE

11.1.2.1   HYPOTHESES

The chi-square test may be used to test for independence of attributes.
   That is,
   H_0: The two attributes are independent.

11.1.2.2   RXK CONTINGENCY TABLE

The $r \times k$ contingency table has r rows and c columns as shown below:

r × k Contingency Table

variable2 / variable1	category 1	category 2	-	category k	Total
category 1	O_{11}	O_{12}		O_{1k}	$O_{1.}$
category 2	O_{21}	O_{22}		O_{2k}	$O_{2.}$
-					
category r	O_{r1}	O_{r2}		O_{rk}	$O_{r.}$
Total	$O_{.1}$	$O_{.2}$		$O_{.k}$	n

11.1.2.3 TEST STATISTIC

It is given by,

$$\chi^2 = \sum \frac{(O_{ij} - e_{ij})^2}{e_{ij}} = \sum \frac{O_{ij}^2}{e_{ij}} - n \text{ with df} = (r-1)(c-1)$$

Where,

$$e_{ij} = \frac{O_i O_j}{n}$$

Example: A classification according to religion and diagnostic categories of 337 psychiatric patients is given in the following table (figures in the bracket are expected frequencies).

Disorder/ religion	Schizophrenia	Affective disorder	Neurotic disorder	Total
Hindu	109 (102.7)	114 (115.1)	56 (61.3)	279
Muslim	8 (16.2)	22 (18.1)	14 (9.7)	44
Christian	7 (5.2)	3 (5.8)	4 (3.1)	14
Total	124	139	74	337

For this data,

$$\chi^2 = \left(\frac{109^2}{102.7} + \frac{114^2}{115.1} \ldots + \frac{4^2}{3.1} \right) - 337 = 347.034 - 337 = 10.03$$

$$df = (3-1)(3-1) = 4$$

The expected frequencies are calculated based on the null hypothesis that the two attributes are independent. For example, the expected frequency for Hindu schizophrenia is calculated as follows:

$$e_{11} = (279 \times 124)/337 = 102.7$$

Since the calculated value is more than the table value of $\chi^2 = 9.49$ at df = 4, we reject the null hypothesis ($P<0.01$, highly significant).

11.1.3 CHI-SQUARE TESTS: 2x2 CONTINGENCY TABLE

11.1.3.1 HYPOTHESES

The chi-square can be used to test whether two binary attributes are independent or not.

11.1.3.2 2 × 2 CONTINGENCY TABLE

The 2×2 contingency table has 2 rows and 2 columns as shown below:

2×2 Contingency Table

Variable 2/variable1	Category 1	Category 2	Total
Category 1	a	b	(a + b)
Category 2	c	d	(c + d)
Total	(a + c)	(b + d)	n

11.1.3.3 TEST STATISTIC

It is given by

$$\chi^2 = \frac{n(ad-bc)^2}{(a+b)(c+d)(a+c)(b+d)} \text{ with df} = 1$$

Example: The classification according to sex and marital status of the 40 patients (data in Appendix I) is as given below:

Marital status/sex	Single	Married	Total
Male	14	10	24
Female	7	9	16
	21	19	Total

For this data,

$$\chi^2 = \frac{40\ (14 \times 9 - 10 \times 7)^2}{24 \times 16 \times 21 \times 19} = \frac{40\ (126 - 70)^2}{24 \times 16 \times 21 \times 19} = 0.82, \text{ with df} = 1$$

Since the calculated value is less than the table value of $\chi^2 = 3.841$, with df = 1, we accept the null hypothesis.

11.1.4   CHI-SQUARE TESTS: 2xK CONTINGENCY TABLE

11.1.4.1   HYPOTHESES

The chi-square test can be used to test whether the two attributes are independent or not.

11.1.4.2   2×K CONTINGENCY TABLE

The 2×k contingency table has 2 rows and k columns as shown below:

2×k Contingency Table

Variable2/variable1	Category1	Category 2	-	Category k	Total
Category 1	X_1	X_2		X_k	X
Category 2	Y_1	Y_2		Y_k	Y
Total	Z_1	Z_2		Z_k	Z

11.1.4.3 TEST STATISTIC

It is given by

$$\chi^2 = \frac{Z^2}{XY}\left(\frac{X_1^2}{Z_1} + \frac{X_2^2}{Z_2} + \ldots + \frac{X_k^2}{Z_k}\right) - \frac{ZX}{Y} \text{ with df} = (k-1)$$

Example: A classification according to type of service and religion of 500 psychiatric patients registered at NIMHANS hospital is as presented below:

Religion/admission status	Hindu	Muslim	Christian	Total
In-patients	133(32.8)	14(21.2)	11(39.3)	158(31.6)
Out-patients	273(67.2)	52(78.8)	17(60.7)	342(68.4)
Total	406(100)	66(100)	28(100)	500(100)

For this data,

$$\chi^2 = \frac{500^2}{158 \times 342}\left(\frac{133^2}{406} + \frac{14^2}{66} + \frac{11^2}{28}\right) - \frac{500 \times 158}{342} = 4.39 \text{ with df} = (k-1)$$

Since the calculated value is less than the table value of chi-square at 2 df (5.99), we accept the null hypothesis ($P>0.05$, not significant).

11.1.5 TESTS OF SIGNIFICANCE OF INDIVIDUAL CELL FREQUENCIES

11.1.5.1 HYPOTHESES

This is the identification of significantly high/low frequencies of individual cells in a contingency table.

11.1.5.2 CONTINGENCY TABLE

The tests of significance of individual cell frequencies are carried out for contingency table of any dimension.

11.1.5.3   TEST STATISTICS

It consists in computing adjusted standardized residuals (Z_{ij}) for each cell frequency in the contingency table. Thus, the test statistics are given by

$$Z_{ij} = \frac{\epsilon_{ij}}{\sqrt{\text{var}(\epsilon_{ij})}}$$

where the standardized residuals (ϵ_{ij}) are given by

$$\epsilon_{ij} = \frac{(o_{ij} - e_{ij})}{\sqrt{e_{ij}}}$$

$$\text{Var}(\epsilon_{ij}) = (1 - p_i)(1 - p_j)$$

where p_i and p_j are the proportions of the marginal totals of the ij-th cell. The ϵ_{ij} are called standardized residuals of the ij-th cell. When the variables forming the contingency table are independent, the Z_{ij} are approximately normally distributed with mean 0 and variance 1.

Example: The observed frequencies and the expected frequencies (in the brackets) of the 40 patients (data in Appendix I) classified according to sex and marital status is given below:

Sex	Single	Married	Total
Male	14 (12.6)	10 (11.4)	24
Female	7 (8.4)	9 (7.6)	16
Total	21	19	40

The residuals ($O_{ij} - e_{ij}$) are given in the following table.

Sex	Single	Married	Total
Male	1.4	−1.4	0
Female	−1.4	1.4	0
Total	0	0	0

The standardized residuals are calculated and presented in the following table.

Sex	Single	Married
Male	0.39	−0.41
Female	−0.48	0.51

Finally, the adjusted standardized residuals Z_{ij} are computed as shown in the following table:

Sex	Single	Married
Male	0.9	−0.9
Female	−0.9	0.9

11.1.6   ONE-SAMPLE RUN TEST

11.1.6.1   HYPOTHESES

The run test is applied to test whether the sequence of events in a sample is at random. Thus, it is a randomization test.

11.1.6.2   SEQUENCE OF EVENTS

The test is based on the number of runs which a sample exhibits, the number of objects in one category (n_1), and the number of objects in another category (n_2). A run is defined as a success of identical symbols thatare followed and proceed by different symbols or no symbol at all.

11.1.6.3   TEST STATISTIC

The test statistic is given by

$$Z = \frac{|r - \mu_r|}{\sigma_r}$$

where $\mu_r = \frac{2n_1 n_2}{n_1 + n_2} + 1$

$$\sigma_r = \sqrt{\frac{2n_1n_2(2n_1n_2 - n_1 - n_2)}{(n_1 + n_2)^2(n_1 + n_2 - 1)}}$$

Too many or two small number of runs do not support randomness.

Example: The 40 patients (data in Appendix I) were registered in the following order of males (M) and females (F):

M FFF MM F MM F M FFF MM F MMMMMMMMM FFF MM F MMMM F M FF

For this data,
Number of males $(n_1) = 24$
Number of females $(n_2) = 16$
Number of runs $(r) = 18$
Hence,

$$\mu_r = \frac{2 \times 24 \times 16}{24 + 16} + 1 = 19.2 + 1 = 20.2$$

$$\sigma_r = \sqrt{\frac{(2 \times 24 \times 16)(2 \times 24 \times 16 - 24 - 16)}{(24 + 16)^2(24 + 16 - 1)}} = \sqrt{8.96} = 2.993$$

$$Z = \frac{|18 - 20.2|}{2.993} = \frac{2.2}{2.993} = 0.735$$

Since the calculated value is less than 1.96, we accept the null hypotheses that the sequence of occurrence of males and females is at random.

11.2   TWO INDEPENDENT SAMPLE NON-PARAMETRIC TESTS

11.2.1   MEDIAN TEST

The median test may be used when the null hypothesis states that the two groups are from population with the same median. This method is applicable whenever the scores of the two groups are in at least an ordinal scale. To perform the median test, we first determine the median score of the combined group. Then, we dichotomize both sets of scores at that combined median. Then, the procedure is to prepare a 2×2 contingency table and apply the chi-square test of significance.

11.2.2 MANN–WHITNEY U-TEST

11.2.2.1 HYPOTHESES

The Mann–Whitney U-test is used to test whether two independent groups have been drawn from the same population. Thus, it is equivalent to the independent sample t-test.

11.2.2.2 MANN–WHITNEY U-TEST TABLE

The method consists in combining the two samples and arranges the observations in order of magnitude. Then, assign ranks to the combined observations from 1 to $(n_1 + n_2)$.

11.2.2.3 TEST STATISTIC

Now, the test statistic is given by

$$Z = \frac{|U - \mu_U|}{\sigma_u}$$

where $U = n_1 n_2 + \dfrac{n_1(n_1 + 1)}{2} - R_1$

R_1 is the sum of the ranks of the first group.

$$\mu_u = \frac{n_1 n_2}{2}$$

$$\sigma_u = \sqrt{\frac{n_1 n_2 (n_1 + n_2 + 1)}{12}}$$

Example: Let us suppose that the marks scored in a test by ten randomly selected students from two departments are given below. We wish to test whether the marks scored by the students in the two departments are the same.

Department 1	Department 2
4	9
2	7
3	8
0	5
6	11

For this data, the scores are converted as ranks as shown below:

Department 1	Department 2
4	9
2	7
3	8
1	5
6	10
16	39

Here,

$R_1 = 16$

$U = (5 \times 5) + \dfrac{5(5+1)}{2} - 16 = 25 + 15 - 16 = 24$

$\mu_u = \dfrac{5 \times 5}{2} = 12.5$

$\sigma_u = \sqrt{\dfrac{5 \times 5(5+5+1)}{12}} = 4.787$

Hence,

$Z = \dfrac{24 - 12.5}{4.787} = \dfrac{11.5}{4.787} = 2.402$

Since, the calculated value is more than 1.96, we reject the null hypotheses of randomness ($P < 0.05$, significant).

11.3   TWO-RELATED SAMPLE NON-PARAMETRIC TESTS

11.3.1   McNEMAR'S TEST

11.3.1.1   HYPOTHESES

The McNemar's test is used when the researcher involved in hypotheses that there is change after the treatment. This test of significance is used when both the variables under study are measured in nominal scale.

11.3.1.2   McNEMAR'S TEST TABLE

The researcher sets up a four-fold table of frequencies to represent first and second sets of responses from the same individual. A typical 2×2 McNemar's test table is given below, where fail and pass are used to signify different responses.

2×2 McNemar's test table

		After	
		Pass	**Fail**
Before	fail	A	B
	pass	C	D

11.3.1.3   TEST STATISTIC

Now, the test statistic is given by

$$\chi^2 = \frac{(A - D)^2}{(A + D)} \text{ with df} = 1.$$

Example: Let us suppose that the results of a test of 36 students before giving the teaching program and the results after taking the teaching program are given in the following table. We wish to test whether there is a significant effect of the training program.

		After		Total
		Pass	Fail	
Before	Fail	16	2	18
	Pass	14	4	18
	Total	30	6	36

$$\chi^2 = (16 - 4)^2/(16 + 4) = 144/20 = 7.20, \text{ with df} = 1$$

Since the calculated value is more than the table value of $\chi^2 = 6.63$, with df = 1 at 1 percent level of significance, we reject the null hypotheses ($P < 0.01$, highly significant). Hence, there is a significant effect of the teaching program.

11.3.2   SIGN TEST

11.3.2.1   HYPOTHESES

The sign test is used when the researcher involves in hypothesis that there is change after the treatment. This test is applied when the data on a variable have underlying continuity but which can be measured in only a very gross way.

11.3.2.2   SIGN TEST TABLE

The sign test uses plus and minus signs rather than quantitative measures as its data. The method consists in focusing on the direction of the difference between every pair of the observations and record plus sign when the other values is less than the value before giving the treatment, and minus sign otherwise.

11.3.2.3   TEST STATISTIC

Now, the test statistic is given by

$$Z = \frac{|x - 0.5n|}{0.5\sqrt{n}}$$

where n is the number of observations

x is the number of plus signs

Example: Let us suppose that the results of 36 students before taking the teaching program and the results of the students after taking the teaching program are given: it is found that 31 students have improved. We wish to test whether there is a significant effect (improvement) of the teaching program.

$$Z = \frac{|31 - 0.5 \times 36|}{0.5\sqrt{36}} = \frac{13}{3} = 4.33$$

Since the calculated value is more than 2.58, the null hypothesis is rejected ($P<0.01$, highly significant). That is, there is a significant effect of the teaching program.

11.4   K-INDEPENDENT SAMPLE NON-PARAMETRIC TESTS

11.4.1   EXTENDED MEDIAN TEST

This is an extension of the median test in which there are more than two groups in the data for this test, and the researcher is interested to test whether these groups are from populations with the same median. The requisite 2×k contingency table has to be prepared, and the chi-square test of significance has to be applied.

11.4.2   KRUSHKAL–WALLIS *H*-TEST

11.4.2.1   HYPOTHESES

This test that is based on ranks is to test whether the *k*-samples are from the same population.

11.4.2.2   KRUSHKAL–WALLIS H-TEST TABLE

In this test, each of the n observations is replaced by ranks. That is, all the scores from all of the k-samples combined are ranked in a single series. The smallest score is replaced by rank 1, the next to smallest by rank 2, and the largest score by rank n. Here, n is the total number of independent observations in the k-samples. Then, the sum of the ranks in each sample (column) is found. To test whether these sum of ranks are so desperate that they are not likely to have come from samples that were all drawn from the same population.

11.4.2.3   TEST STATISTIC

Now, the test statistic is given by

$$H = \frac{12}{n(n+1)} \sum \frac{R_j^2}{n_j} - 3\,(n+1)$$

The H follows approximate chi-square with df $= (k - 1)$
where k is the number of samples (groups)
n is the number of cases in all the samples combined
n_j is the number of cases in the jth sample
R_j is the sum of the ranks in the jth sample
Example: Let us suppose that the marks scored by 15 randomly selected students from three departments are as given in the following table.

Department 1	Department 2	Department 3
4	9	14
2	7	12
3	8	13
0	5	10
6	11	16

We wish to test whether the scores from the three departments are same. The ranks of the observations (scores) in the three departments combined are given in the following table.

	Department 1	Department 2	Department 3
	4	9	14
	2	7	12
	3	8	13
	1	5	10
	6	11	15
Sum of ranks	16	40	64
Mean ranks	3.2	8.0	12.8

For this data,

$$H= \frac{12}{(15 \times 16)} \left(\frac{16^2}{5} + \frac{40^2}{5} + \frac{64^2}{5} \right) - 3 \times 6 = 59.52 - 48 = 11.52$$

with df $= (3 - 1) = 2$

Since the calculated value is more than the table value of χ^2 (2) $= 9.21$, we reject the null hypothesis ($P < 0.01$, highly significant).

11.5   K-RELATED SAMPLE NON-PARAMETRIC TESTS

11.5.1   COCHRAN Q-TEST

11.5.1.1   HYPOTHESES

This is an extension of the McNemar's test in which there are more than two related samples for Cochran Q-test. This provides a method for testing whether three or more matched sets of frequencies or proportion differ significantly among themselves. This test is particularly suitable when the data are dichotomized ordinal information.

11.5.1.2   COCHRAN Q-TEST TABLE

A typical Cochran Q-test table is as given below:

Cochran Q-test table

Serial number	Repeat 1	Repeat 2	Repeat k	Total
1				L_1
2				L_2
-				-
n				L_n
Total (G)	G_1	G_2	G_k	

11.5.1.3 TEST STATISTIC

A typical $n \times k$ Cochran Q-test table is given below (pass, 1; fail, 0) in which students are tested in three occasions.

Student	Repeat 1	Repeat 2	Repeat 3
1	1	1	1
2	0	1	1
3	0	0	1
4	0	0	1
5	1	1	1

Now, the test statistic is given by

$$Q = \frac{(k-1)\left(k \sum G_j^2 - (G_j)^2\right)}{k \sum L_i - \sum L_i^2}$$

The Q follows approximate χ^2 with df $= (k-1)$

where k is the number of repetitions (conditions)

G_j is the sum of the jth column

L_i is the sum of the ith row

Example: Let us suppose that the scores obtained on three repetitions of five students are as given in the following table.

Student	Repeat 1	Repeat 2	Repeat 3	L_i	L_i^2
1	1	1	1	3	9
2	0	1	1	2	4
3	0	0	1	1	1
4	0	0	1	1	1
5	1	1	1	3	9
G_j	2	3	5	10	24
G_j^2	4	9	25		38

$$Q = \frac{2(3 \times 38 - 10^2)}{(3 \times 10 - 24)} = \frac{2(114 - 100)}{(30 - 24)} = \frac{28}{6} = 4.67 \text{ with df} = (3-1) = 2$$

Since the calculated value is less than the Table value of $\chi^2 = 5.99$ with df = 2, we accept the null hypotheses ($P > 0.05$, not significant). That is, the teaching program has no significant effect.

11.5.2   FRIEDMAN TEST

11.5.2.1   HYPOTHESES

The Friedman test of significance is used when the researcher has the hypothesis that the k-related sample has come from different populations with respect to mean ranks. The test is applicable when the measurement of the variable are expressed as ranks.

11.5.2.2   FRIEDMAN TEST TABLE

It is given by,
Friedman test table

Serial number	Rank (repeat 1)	Rank (repeat 2)	-	Rank (repeat k)
1	-	-	-	-
2	-	-	-	--
-	-	-	-	-
n	-	-	-	-
Sum	R_1	R_2	-	R_k

The data are given in a two-way table having n rows and k columns. The rows represent the various subjects or matched set of subjects and the columns represent the various conditions. The data of the test are ranks. The scores in each row are ranked separately with k conditions being studied, the ranks in any row ranked from 1 to k.

11.5.2.3   TEST STATISTIC

Now, the teat statistic is given by

$$\chi^2 = \frac{12}{nk(k+1)} \sum R_j^2 - 3n(k+1) \text{ with df} = (k-1)$$

where n is the number of rows (patients, subjects)

k is the number of columns (conditions)

R_j is the sum of ranks of the jth column

Example: Let us suppose that the marks scored by five students (on a teaching program) in three consecutively conducted tests are given below. We wish to test whether there is a significant improvement of teaching program in repeated tests.

Student	Repeat 1	Repeat 2	Repeat 3
1	4	7	10
2	2	4	7
3	3	1	8
4	0	3	6
5	6	5	4

The requisite computation table (ranks of the marks) is as given below:

Student	Rank (repeat 1)	Rank (repeat 2)	Rank (repeat 3)
1	1	2	3
2	1	2	3
3	2	1	3

Student	Rank (repeat 1)	Rank (repeat 2)	Rank (repeat 3)
4	1	2	3
5	3	2	1
sum	8	9	13
mean	1.6	1.8	3.6

Now,

$$\chi^2 = \frac{12}{(5 \times 3 \times 4)} (8^2 + 9^2 + 13^2) - (3 \times 5 \times 4) = \frac{1}{5}(64 + 81 + 169) - 60 = 2.80,$$

with df $= (3 - 1) = 2$

Since, the calculated value is less than the table value of $\chi^2 = 5.99$, with df $= 2$, we accept the null hypothesis ($P > 0.05$, not significant). That is, there is no significant improvement in the repeated administration of the program.

KEYWORDS

- **Contingency table**
- **Non-parametric tests**
- **Test statistics**

CHAPTER 12

CORRELATION ANALYSIS AND REGRESSION ANALYSIS

CONTENTS

12.1   TWO-QUANTITATIVE VARIABLES CORRELATION COEFFICIENTS

12.1.1   SCATTER DIAGRAM

The primary step in correlation analysis is to present the bivariate data (two-variable data) on a graph sheet and grasp the type of relationship. Such a graphical representation is known as scatter diagram or dot diagram. The scatter diagrams showing different types of relationship are given in Figure 12.1.

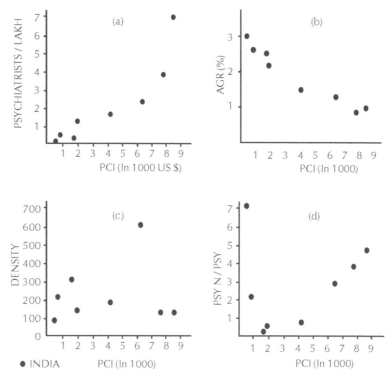

FIGURE 12.1   The dot diagram (a) shows the positive linear relationship between per capita income (PCI) and the number of psychiatrists per one lakh population of eight countries. The dot diagram (b) shows the negative linear relationship between PCI and annual growth rate (AGR) of population. The dot diagram (c) shows no relationship between PCI and the density of population. The dot diagram (d) shows curvilinear relationship between PCI and number of psychiatric nurses per psychiatrist manpower.

12.1.2 PEARSON CORRELATION COEFFICIENT

We limit our study to linear relationship and the theory built upon this assumption is known as linear or simple correlation. The product movement correlation coefficient or Pearson correlation coefficient measures such relationship. It is given by

$$r = \frac{\sum xy - n\bar{x}\,\bar{y}}{\sqrt{\left(\sum x^2 - n\bar{x}^2\right)\left(\sum y^2 - n\bar{y}^2\right)}}$$

The r lies between -1 and 1.

$r = 1$ means perfect positive linear relationship

$r = -1$ means perfect negative linear relationship

$r = 0$ means no linear relationship

The standard error of r is given by

$$SE\,(r) = \sqrt{\frac{1 - r^2}{(n-2)}}$$

12.1.2.1 TEST OF SIGNIFICANCE

The procedures for testing a population correlation coefficient (ρ) equals zero is given below:

H_0: $\rho = 0$ against H_1: $\rho \neq 0$

The test statistic is given by

$$t = \frac{r\sqrt{n-2}}{\sqrt{1-r^2}} \text{ with df} = (n-2)$$

Example: Let us suppose that the marks scored in mathematics (x), and the marks scored in statistics (y) by a group of five students are given in the following table.

Student	Maths (x)	Statistics (y)
1	4	7
2	2	4
3	3	1
4	0	3
5	6	5

For this data, the computation table is given below:

Student	(x)	y	x^2	y^2	xy
1	4	7	16	49	28
2	2	4	4	16	8
3	3	1	9	1	3
4	0	3	0	9	0
5	6	5	36	25	30
Total	15	20	65	100	69

Now,

$$r = \frac{69 - 5 \times 3 \times 4}{\sqrt{(65 - 5 \times 3^2)(100 - 5 \times 4^2)}} = \frac{69 - 60}{\sqrt{20 \times 20}} = \frac{9}{20} = 0.45$$

12.1.2.2   TEST OF SIGNIFICANCE

$$t = \frac{0.45\sqrt{5-2}}{\sqrt{1-0.45^2}} = \frac{0.45\sqrt{3}}{\sqrt{1-0.2025}} = 0.872, \text{ with df} = (5-2) = 3$$

Since the calculated value is less than the table value of $t(3) = 3.18$, the null hypothesis is accepted ($P > 0.05$, not significant).

12.2   RANK CORRELATION COEFFICIENTS

12.2.1   SPEARMAN RANK CORRELATION COEFFICIENT

The Spearman rank correlation coefficient is derived for the situation in which the observed values of both the variables are expressed as ranks. It is given by

$$r_s = 1 - \frac{6 \sum d_i^2}{n(n^2 - 1)}$$

The d_i is the difference between the ranks of the two variables of the ith individual. The r_s lies between -1 and 1.

Example: Let us calculate the Spearman rank correlation coefficient for the data used to demonstrate the Pearson correlation coefficient. The computation table is as given below:

Student	x	y	Ranks of x	Ranks of y	d_i	d_i^2
1	4	7	4	5	−1	1
2	2	4	2	3	−1	1
3	3	1	3	1	2	4
4	0	3	1	2	−1	1
5	6	5	5	4	1	1
Total						8

Now,

$$r_s = 1 - \frac{6 \times 8}{5\,(5^2 - 1)} = 1 - \frac{6 \times 8}{5 \times 24} = 0.60$$

12.3 TWO-QUALITATIVE VARIABLES CORRELATION COEFFICIENTS

12.3.1 CONTINGENCY COEFFICIENT

The first step in calculating the contingency coefficient is to present the data in a contingency table. The contingency coefficient is computed for the data in which both the variables are measured in nominal level. It is given by

$$CC = \sqrt{\frac{\chi^2}{\chi^2 + n}}$$

where χ^2 is the chi-square value. The CC lies between 0 and less than 1.

Example: The 2 × 2 contingency table for calculating the CC for sex and marital status of 40 patients (data in Appendix I) is given below:

Sex	Single	Married	Total
Male	14	10	24
Female	7	9	16
Total	21	19	40

For this data,

$$CC = \sqrt{\frac{0.819}{0.819 + 40}} = 0.142$$

12.3.2 PHI COEFFICIENT

The phi-correlation coefficient is computed for the data in which both the variables being correlated are genuine dichotomous, and the classes are separated by a real gap between them. In order to compute phi-coefficient, the 2 × 2 contingency table has to be prepared. The phi-coefficient is given by (with usual notations),

$$\emptyset = \frac{(ad - bc)}{\sqrt{(a+b)(c+d)(a+c)(b+d)}}$$

where a, b, c, and d are the frequencies in the 2 × 2 contingency table. The Ø lies between −1 and 1.

Example: Association between sex and marital status of the 40 patients used to demonstrate the contingency coefficient is calculated as follows:

$$\emptyset = \frac{(14 \times 9 - 10 \times 7)}{\sqrt{24 \times 16 \times 21 \times 19)}} = 0.142$$

12.4 MEASURES OF RELATIVE RISKS

In observational longitudinal studies such as retrospective studies and prospective studies, we attempt to measure the relative risk of various risk factors on several diseases/disorders. For analysis of such data, the 2×2 risk and disease table has to be prepared as shown below.

		Disease		Total
		Present	Absent	
Risk	Present	a	b	(a + b)
	Absent	c	d	(c + d)

12.4.1 RISK DIFFERENCE

The risk difference is defined as follows:

RD = (risk in the exposed group-risk in the normal group)

$$= \left(\frac{a}{a+b}\right) - \left(\frac{c}{c+d}\right)$$

The RD lies between −1 and 1.

12.4.2 RISK RATIO

The risk ratio is defined as follows:

$$RR = \frac{\text{Incidence of the disease among exposed}}{\text{Incidence of the disease among non-exposed}}$$

$$= \left(\frac{a}{a+b}\right) / \left(\frac{c}{c+d}\right)$$

The RR lies between zero and infinity.

12.4.3 ODDS RATIO

The odds ratio is defined as follows:

$$OR = \frac{\text{Odds that exposed individuals will have disease}}{\text{Odds that non-exposed individuals will have disease}}$$

$$= \left(\frac{a}{b}\right) / \left(\frac{c}{d}\right) = \frac{ad}{bc}$$

The OR lies between zero and infinity.

OR < 1 means the exposed is protected

OR = 1 means there is no effect

OR > 1 means the exposed is harmful

Thus, OR indicates the number of times the risk is harmful in comparison with the normal.

12.4.4   TEST OF SIGNIFICANCE OF ODDS RATIO

The procedure for test of significance of OR equals 1 is given by,

H_0: OR = 1 against H_1: OR ≠ 1

We have the transformation, $\lambda = l_n$ (OR)

Now, H_0: $\lambda = 0$ against H_1: $\lambda \neq 0$

The test statistic is given by

$$Z = \frac{\hat{\lambda}}{\sqrt{\text{var}(\hat{\lambda})}}$$

where $\hat{\lambda}$ is based on the sample values.

$$\text{Var}(\hat{\lambda}) = \left(\frac{1}{a} + \frac{1}{b} + \frac{1}{c} + \frac{1}{d} \right)$$

Example: Let us suppose that the data are given in the following 2 × 2 risk and disease table.

		Disease		Total
		present	absent	
Risk	present	13	9	22
	absent	1	13	14

For this data,

RD = $\frac{13}{22} - \frac{1}{14}$ = 0.591 − 0.071 = 0.520

RR = $\frac{13}{22} \big/ \frac{1}{14}$ = 0.591/0.071 = 8.27

OR = $\frac{13}{9} \big/ \frac{1}{13}$ = (13 × 13)/9 = 169/9 = 18.78

The test of significance of OR is carried out as follows:

$$\lambda = l_n (OR) = l_n (18.78) = 2.933$$

$$\text{Var}(\hat{\lambda}) = (\tfrac{1}{13} + \tfrac{1}{9} + \tfrac{1}{1} + \tfrac{1}{13}) = 0.0769 + 0.1111 + 1.0000 + 0.0769 = 1.265$$

$$Z = \frac{2.933}{\sqrt{1.265}} = 2.61$$

Since the calculated value is more than 2.58, we reject the null hypotheses ($P < 0.01$, highly significant)

12.5   REGRESSION ANALYSIS

The main purpose of regression analysis is to predict the value of the dependent variable (y) when the value of the independent variable (x) is given. The analysis describes the dependency of a variable on independent variables, suggests possible cause-and-effect relationship between factors, and explains some of the variation of the dependent variable by the independent variables by using the latter as a control. For example, the studies such as (1) dose of amytryptaline on the reduction of depression and (2) effect of urbanization on the increase of prevalence of neurotic disorder of a defined population.

12.5.1   LINEAR REGRESSION ANALYSIS

In linear regression analysis (one-independent variable), a straight line passing through the data in dot diagram is to be fitted.

12.5.1.1   FITTING LINEAR REGRESSION EQUATION

The straight line equation is given by

$$y = a + bx$$

where a is the intercept
b is the slope of the straight line called regression coefficient
The parameters a and b are determined in such a way that the sum of squares of deviations of the observed values from their regression esti-

mates is minimum. This is a typical problem in differential calculus. The values for a and b are given by

$$a = \bar{y} - b\,\bar{x}$$

$$b = \frac{\sum xy - n\bar{x}\,\bar{y}}{\sum x^2 - n\bar{x}^2}$$

Hence,

$$\hat{y} = a + bx$$

where $\hat{y}$ is the predicted value of the dependent variable for the given value of the independent variable x.

Example: Let us suppose that the dosage (x) and the improvement score (y) of a group of 5 students are given below:

Patient	Dosage	Improvement
1	4	7
2	2	4
3	3	1
4	0	3
5	6	5

For this data,

$$b = \frac{69 - 5 \times 3 \times 4}{65 - 5 \times 3^2} = \frac{9}{20} = 0.45$$

$$a = 4 - 0.45 \times 3 = 4 - 1.35 = 2.65$$

Hence, the regression equation is given by

$$\hat{y} = 2.65 + 0.45x$$

That is, the predicted improvement score $= 2.65 + 0.45 \times$ dose

Patient	Dosage (x)	Improvement (y)	Improvement ($\hat{y}$) estimate	Residuals ($y - \hat{y}$)
1	4	7	4.45	2.55
2	2	4	3.55	0.45
3	3	1	4.00	−3.00
4	0	3	2.65	0.35
5	6	5	5.35	−0.35
Total	15	20	20.00	0

The linear regression line is given in Figure 12.2.

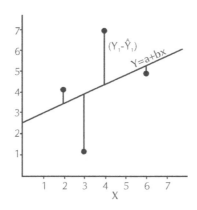

FIGURE 12.2   Dot diagram showing regression line of y on x.

Let us suppose that a patient is given a dose 1. Then, his predicted improvement score is determined as follows:

$\hat{y} = 2.65 + 0.45 \times 1 = 2.65 + 0.45 = 3.10$, approximately equals to 3

12.5.2 LOGISTIC REGRESSION ANALYSIS

The logistic regression is used to predict a discrete outcome. If the dependent variable has only two outcomes, the method is called binary logistic regression. If there are more than two outcomes associated with the dependent variable, the method is called multinomial logistic regression. The logistic regression computes the log (natural) odds for a particular outcome. The odds of an outcome are given by the ratio of the probability of it happening and not happening. That is,

$$\text{Odds} = \frac{P}{1-P}$$

where P is the probability of an event. We calculate

$$l_n\left(\frac{P}{1-P}\right)$$

The values range from $-\infty$ to ∞. A positive value indicates that odds are in favour of the event and the event is likely to occur, whereas a negative value indicates that odds are against the event and the event is not likely to occur. For establishing model fit, SPSS calculates chi-square values based on log-likelihood values.

KEYWORDS

- Chi-square value
- Contingency table
- Correlation coefficient
- Regression analysis

CHAPTER 13

RELIABILITY ANALYSIS AND VALIDITY ANALYSIS

CONTENTS

13.1   SCALING TECHNIQUES

The simplest way of measuring one's attitude is to ask him to rate his strength by himself. This can be done by constructing a scale by using summated scaling method or equal interval scaling method.

13.1.1   SUMMATED SCALING TECHNIQUE

In this method of measuring one's attitude is by presenting him with a number of attitude statements of varying intensity. The steps involved in construction and administration of summated scale are as follows:

Step 1: About 50 items are selected from the bank of items measuring the attitude/trait. These items must be valid and reliable.

Step 2: About 50 percent of the items are positively worded and the remaining 50 percent of the items are negatively worded.

Step 3: About 3–7 response categories ranging from low to high intensity of each item are to be adapted.

Step 4: The positively worded items must be measured in one order and then negatively worded items must be measured in the reverse order.

Step 5: The respondents are asked to tick the response categories for each item in the scale.

Step 6: We sum the scores of these items to portray their position of intensity.

Step 7: Transform the scores into ordinal level to facilitate appropriate analysis.

13.1.2   EQUAL-INTERVAL SCALING TECHNIQUE

In equal-interval scaling (Thurstone scaling), the respondents are presented with a hypothetical range of attitudes from extreme favourableness to extreme unfavourableness graphically or pictorially. The steps involved in construction and administration of Thurstone scale are as follows:

Step 1: About 50 items are selected from the bank of items.

Step 2: About 20 judges are asked to sort out these items into about 7 categories ranging from high to low intensity.

Step 3: The weight of each item is based on the average of the categories into which it has been sorted out by the judges.

Step 4: About 20 items are selected for use in the final questionnaire.

Step 5: The respondents are asked to select two or three items that best reflect their sentiments toward the psychological objects in question.

Step 6: We calculate the mean of these items to portray their position along the continuum of intensity.

Step 7: The Thurstone scaling measures lend themselves to interval level of measurement.

13.2   RELIABILITY ANALYSIS

Reliability is the consistency of a set of measurements or of a measuring instrument, often used to describe a test. There are several general classes of reliability estimates: test–retest reliability that includes intrarater reliability, internal consistency reliability, inter-rater reliability, and inter-method reliability.

13.2.1   *TEST–RETEST RELIABILITY OF SCALES*

It is the variation in measurements taken by a single person or instrument on the same items and under the same conditions. Thus, the test–retest method consists in submitting a group of individuals to a particular test and compiling their respective scores. After some time, the same test is repeated on the same group of individuals, and their scores are noted down. Then, the correlation between the two sets of related scores is obtained to measure the reliability of the test.

If the test is repeated immediately after the first, then the scores are likely to be improved on account of the memory effect, practice, and confidence. If sufficient time is given, then some other factors may come in such as growth in case of children, which may increase the scores. This method is generally used to measure the reliability of speed tests where speed is an important criterion. It is appropriate when the test is heterogeneous in the sense that different parts measure different traits (multidimensional scaling).

13.2.2 UNI-DIMENSIONAL SCALING

When items are used to form a scale, they need to have interval consistency. The items should all measure the same thing; therefore, they should be correlated with one another.

13.2.2.1 CRONBACH'S ALPHA

A useful coefficient for assessing interval consistency is Cronbach's alpha. It is given by

$$\text{Cronbach's alpha} = \frac{k\bar{c}}{(k-1)\bar{c}+\bar{v}}$$

where $\bar{c}$ is the mean of covariances

$\bar{v}$ is the mean of variances

k is the number of items

Example: Let us suppose that the rating scores on services rendered by a mental health institute (hospital) as rated by 5 raters on 3 items are given below:

Rater	Item 1	Item 2	Item 3
1	4	7	10
2	2	4	7
3	3	1	8
4	0	3	6
5	6	5	4

For this data, the variance–covariance matrix is given below:

Items	Item 1	Item 2	Item 3
Item 1	4	1.8	−0.6
Item 2	1.8	4	0.8
Item 3	−0.6	0.8	4

$$\text{Cronbach's alpha} = \frac{3 \times 0.667}{(2 \times 0.667)+4} = 0.375$$

13.2.3 INTERNAL CONSISTENCY RELIABILITY OF SCALES

It assesses the consistency of results across items included in a test. The internal consistency reliability is usually measured by split-half method or the method of rational equivalence. These methods are appropriate for power test in which all examiners have time to furnish.

13.2.3.1 SPLIT-HALF METHOD

The split-half method consists in breaking the original test into two equivalent halves and computing the correlation coefficient (r_{hh}) between the scores in half tests. Then, the reliability coefficient for the whole test is determined in terms of self-correlation of the half tests by using Spearman–Brown prophecy formula,

$$r_{tt} = \frac{2 r_{hh}}{1 + r_{hh}}$$

In case of power test, the test items are arranged in increasing order of difficulty and then splitting them into two equivalent halves with odd and even numbered items provide a unique estimate of reliability.

13.2.4 INTER-RATER RELIABILITY OF CONCEPTS

Even if a concept such as schizophrenia is validated by certain genetic, biochemical, psychological, course or treatment variables, the inter-rater reliability assessment of such a concept is required to assume communicative value or to provide scientific evaluation.

13.2.4.1 TWO-RATERS AND DICHOTOMOUS RATINGS

The first step in the analysis of two-raters and dichotomous ratings is to present the data in a 2×2 dichotomous ratings table as shown below:

Rater A	Rater B	
	Agreed	Not-agreed
Agreed	a	b
Not-agreed	c	d

13.2.4.2   KAPPA COEFFICIENT

The inter-rater reliability is measured by using kappa coefficient. It is given by

$$K = \frac{(p_0 - p_c)}{(1 - p_c)}$$

where p_0 is the proportion of the sum of the main diagonal entries
  p_c is the proportion of the sum of the chance number of agreements
  Hence,

$$P_0 = \frac{(a + d)}{(a + b + c + d)}$$

$$p_c = \frac{E(a) + E(d)}{(a + b + c + d)}$$

The kappa coefficient lies between −1 and 1.
$k = 1$ means perfect agreement
$k = 0$ means no agreement
$k = -1$, means perfect disagreement.
Example: Let us suppose that the following data are the result of making diagnosis (schizophrenia or not) by two-raters A and B:

Rater A	Rater B		Total
	Schizophrenia	Non-schizophrenia	
Schizophrenia	40	20	60
Non-Schizophrenia	10	30	40
Total	50	50	100

For this data,

$$p_0 = \frac{(40 + 30)}{100} = 0.70$$

The chance frequency for schizophrenia by both the raters is given by

$$E(\text{schizophrenia and schizophrenia}) = \frac{(50 \times 60)}{100} = 30$$

The chance frequency for non-schizophrenia by both the raters is given by

$$E\,(\text{non-schizophrenia and non-schizophrenia}) = \frac{(50 \times 40)}{100} = 20$$

Hence,

$$p_c = \frac{(30 + 20)}{100} = 0.50$$

$$k = \frac{(0.70 - 0.50)}{(1 - 0.50)} = \frac{0.2}{0.5} = 0.40$$

13.2.4.3   TWO-RATERS AND POLYCHOTOMOUS RATINGS

The two-raters and polychotomous ratings can be dealt with by applying the kappa coefficient (k) as described above.

13.3   VALIDITY ANALYSIS

The validity of a test is the accuracy with which it measures what it is supposed or intended to measure. The validity of a test is determined experimentally by obtaining the correlation coefficient between the test (x) and on some other independent standard test scores (y) called criterion. A criterion may be an objective measure.

13.3.1   VALIDITY CRITERIA

It is difficult to measure validity in practice because of several concepts involved in it.

13.3.1.1   FACE VALIDITY AND CONTENT VALIDITY

The face validity establishes whether the measuring device looks like it is measuring the correct characteristics. The face validity is done by showing the instrument to experts. The content validity refers to the extent to which a measurement reflects the specific intended domain of content. To establish content validity, researchers should first define the entire domain of their study and then assess if the instrument they are using truly represents this domain.

13.3.1.2   PREDICTIVE VALIDITY AND CONCURRENT VALIDITY

The predictive validity means that the measurement should be able to predict other measures of the same thing. For example, if a student is doing well on mathematics examination, he should also do well during his statistics examination. The predictive validity can also be a forecasting validity. The concurrent validity describes the present one.

13.3.1.3   CONSTRUCT VALIDITY AND FACTOR VALIDITY

The construct validity tries to establish an agreement between the measuring instrument and theoretical concepts. To establish construct validity, one must first establish a theoretical relationship and examine the empirical relationship. The factorial validity of a given test is defined by its factor loadings, and these are given by the correlation of the tests with each factor.

13.3.2   VALIDITY INDICES OF SCALE ITEMS

The selected items for a rating scale must be moderately difficult and have good discriminating indices.

13.3.2.1   DIFFICULT INDEX

The difficult index of an item in a scale indicates the proportion of candidates wrongly answered the item. Thus, the difficult index of the ith item is given by

$$Dif(i) = \frac{\text{Number of incorrect answers to the } i^{th} \text{ item}}{\text{Total number of responses to the } i^{th} \text{ item}}$$

The difficult index lies between 0 and 1. All the items in the scale must have moderate difficult indices. They are constructed in such a way that 50 percent of the candidates are expected to answer correctly, since the variation (information) is maximum at $p = 0.50$, which is $pq = 0.25$. That is, as p approximates to 0 or 1, the variance decreases toward the vanishing point.

13.3.2.2   DISCRIMINATION INDEX

The discrimination index of a test item is the power of the item to discriminate between people of favourable attitude and people of unfavourable attitude. The discrimination index of the ith item is given by

$$\text{Dis}(i) = \frac{\begin{array}{c}\text{Number of correct answers} \\ \text{to the } i^{th} \text{ item in the} \\ \text{favourable group}\end{array} - \begin{array}{c}\text{Number of correct answers} \\ \text{to the } i^{th} \text{ item in the} \\ \text{unfavourable group}\end{array}}{\text{Number of cases in the favourable group}}$$

where the favourable group consists of the first 27 percent and the unfavourable group consists of the last 27 percent of the individual arranged in decreasing order of aggregate of marks scored by them. The discrimination index lies between −1 and 1. The Dis (i) is 1 means that a person who passes the ith item would be in the favourable group and a person who fails that item would be in the unfavourable group. The discrimination index is said to be satisfactory if it is more than 0.30.

Example: The marks scored on each of the 5 items measuring the knowledge in statistics by 11 students are tabulated as given below:

Student	Item 1	Item 2	Item 3	Item 4	Item 5	Total
1	1	1	1	1	1	5
2	1	1	1	1	1	5
3	1	1	1	0	1	4
4	1	1	1	0	1	4
5	1	0	1	0	1	3
6	1	0	0	1	1	3
7	1	0	1	0	1	3
8	0	0	1	0	1	2
9	0	0	1	0	1	2
10	0	0	1	0	1	2
11	1	0	0	0	1	2
Total	8	4	9	3	11	35
Dif(i)	.27	0.64	.18	.73	0	
Dis(i)	.67	1.00	.33	.67	0	

Since the difficult index of the 5th item is 0 (far away from 0.50), and its discriminate index is also zero, it is not worth retaining it in the scale.

KEYWORDS

- **Inter-rater reliability**
- **Test–retest method**

CHAPTER 14

SURVIVAL ANALYSIS AND TIME SERIES ANALYSIS

CONTENTS

14.1 SURVIVAL ANALYSIS

The life table techniques are mainly applied in survival analysis, which deal with the expectation of occurrence of phenomenon according to time or the probability of occurrence of the events by time. The life table techniques were originally developed in the field of demography to express the duration of life experienced by a particular group of population during a particular period. The life table techniques may be applied to study the duration of stay of admitted patients in a mental institute (hospital stay tables). They may be applied to follow-up data of specific psychiatric patients maintained with certain specific drug/therapy (clinical life table). In hospital stay table, the admissions, patients remaining in the hospital, and the discharged cases are analogous to the births, living population, and deaths in the demography life table.

14.1.1 COHORT HOSPITAL STAY TABLE TECHNIQUE

The cohort hospital stay table is based on cohort life table techniques. Let us suppose that a group of patients who are admitted in a psychiatric emergency ward on a particular day were followed up in time and noted down how many of them remained at the end of the first day, how many of them remained at the end of the second day, and so on. From this basic data, the other components of cohort hospital stay table are computed as described below:

x: x is the stay in days. It is taken as 0, 1, 2, …. for a complete hospital stay table, and the values of x may be taken like 0, 5, 10, …. and so on for an abridged life table.

l_x: l_x is the basic component. It is the number of patients who stayed up to the end of the xth day.

d_x: The d_x is the number of patients who got discharged between the xth day and the $(x+1)$th day. Thus,

$$d_x = l_x - l_{x+1}$$

L_x: L_x is the number of days stayed by the cohort between the xth day and the $(x+1)$th day. Hence, it is estimated by

$$L_x = l_x - \frac{1}{2} d_x$$

T_x: T_x is the number of days stayed by the cohort beyond the xth day. Thus, it is given by

$$T_x = L_x + L_{x+1} + ...$$

e_x: e_x is the expectation of further duration of stay of a patient who has already stayed for x days. It is estimated by

$$e_x = \frac{T_x}{l_x}$$

Example: Let us suppose that a group of 20 patients who were admitted in an emergency ward on a particular day were followed up in time and noted down how many of them remained at the end of the first day, how many of them remained at the end of the second day, and so on. This data denoted by l_x are given in the following table:

x	0	1	2	3	4	5	6
l_x	20	19	18	11	6	3	1

For this data, the cohort hospital stay table is prepared as shown below:

Cohort hospital stay table

x	l_x	d_x	L_x	T_x	e_x
(1)	(2)	(3)	(4)	(5)	(6)
0	20	1	19.5	68.0	3.4
1	19	1	18.5	48.5	2.6
2	18	7	14.5	30.0	1.7
3	11	5	8.5	15.5	1.4
4	6	3	4.5	7.0	1.2
5	3	2	2.0	2.5	0.8
6	1	1	0.5	0.5	0.5

The examples for calculating various components are as given below:

$d_2 = 18 - 11 = 7$

$L_2 = 18 - 3.5 = 14.5$

$T_2 = 0.5 + 2.0 + 4.5 + 8.5 + 14.5 = 30.0$

$e_2 = 30/18 = 1.7$

14.1.2 CURRENT HOSPITAL STAY TABLE TECHNIQUE

The basic component for a current hospital stay table is the duration of stay (d_x) of a group of patients discharged from the hospital. From this basic data, the other components of current hospital stay table are computed as described in the following table.

x: x is the interval start time in days.

d_x: d_x is the basic component. This is the number of patients discharged in the interval xth and $(x + 1)$th day.

l_x: This is the number of patients entering into the interval xth and $(x + 1)$th day.

$$l_x = l_{(x-1)} - d_{(x-1)}$$

p_x: This is the proportion of patients discharged between the xth and $(x + 1)$th day.

$$p_x = \frac{d_x}{l_x}$$

q_x: This is the proportion of patients staying in the interval xth and $(x + 1)$th day.

$$q_x = 1 - p_x$$

cd_x: This is the cumulative number of patients discharged up to xth day.

$$cd_x = \sum d_x$$

cp_x: This is the cumulative proportion of patients discharged up to the xth day.

$$cp_x = \frac{l_0 - cd_x}{l_0}$$

pd$_x$: This is the probability density of discharge.

$$pd_x = cp_{(x-1)} - cp_x$$

HR$_x$: This is known as hazard ratio. It is given by

$$HR_x = \frac{d_x}{(l_x - 0.5d_x)}$$

Example: Let us suppose that the number of days stayed by 20 patients is given below:

Duration of stay (d_x)	0	1	2	3	4	5	6
Frequency (patients)	1	1	7	5	3	2	1

The current hospital stay table is prepared and presented as shown below:

Current hospital stay table

x	d_x	l_x	p_x	q_x	cd_x	cp_x	pd_x	HR_x
(1)	(2)	(3)	(4)	(5)	(6)	(7)	(8)	(9)
0	1	20	.050	.950	1	.950	.050	.051
1	1	19	.053	.947	2	.900	.050	.054
2	7	18	.389	.611	9	.550	.350	.483
3	5	11	.455	.545	14	.300	.250	.588
4	3	6	.500	.500	17	.150	.150	.667
5	2	3	.667	.333	19	.050	.100	1.000
6	1	1	1.000	.000	20	.000	.050	2.000

Examples for calculating the various components are as given below:

$$l_2 = 20 - 2 = 18$$
$$p_2 = 7/18 = 0.389$$
$$q_2 = 1 - 0.3889 = 0.611$$
$$cd_2 = 1 + 1 + 7 = 9$$
$$cp_2 = (20 - 9)/20 = 0.550$$

$$pd_2 = 0.900 - 0.550 = 0.350$$

$$HR_2 = 7/(18 - 3.5) = 0.483$$

14.2 TIME SERIES ANALYSIS

In many instances, the events behave predictably over time. In such cases, we can use time series forecasting to predict what will happen next. That is, a time series analysis deals with the factors influencing variation of several phenomena according to time and thus aid in forecasting events. A time series is a set of statistical observations arranged in chronological order. That is, time series is a sample of repeated measures of a single variable observed at regular intervals over a period of time. The length of the intervals could be hours, daily, monthly, or yearly. What is most important is that it should be regular. We typically expect to find over or more of the common idealized pattern in a time series, often in combination with one another.

14.2.1 TIME SERIES COMPONENTS

14.2.1.1 TREND

The trend of the time series indicates whether the series increase or decrease. For example, the yearly number of registrations in a newly established mental health institute over a period of 20 years.

14.2.1.2 SEASONAL VARIATION

The seasonal variation represents that portion of a series which may be attributed to the time of the year. For example, (1) the monthly number of registrations in a mental health institute over a period of 20 years and (2) monthly incidence rates of affective disorders in a rural community over a period of 20 years.

14.2.1.3   CYCLICAL COMPONENT

The cyclical component of a time series analysis is a phenomenon that is observed more frequently than the duration of the time series. The phenomena may be attributed to the administrative reforms of the hospital, natural calamity in the surrounding community, etc. For example, the yearly suicides rates in India over a period of 20 years.

14.2.1.4   RANDOM FLUCTUATIONS

The random fluctuations or irregular fluctuations are the movements in the data that cannot be considered as one of the proceeding types.

14.2.2   DECOMPOSITION OF TIME SERIES COMPONENTS

It is rare to find a real time series which is a pure case of just one component. The time series components could be related in any manner, but the relationship is usually considered to be additive. That is, some observation Y is composed of the components given by

$$Y = T + S + C + R$$

14.2.2.1   TREND

The secular trend or linear trend may be determined by fitting a least-square straight line equation to the data. That is,

$$Y = a + bx$$

where x represents the time variable whose values are given serially from 1 to the number of observations.

14.2.2.2   SEASONAL VARIATION

In decomposing of seasonal variation, often the arithmetic means of the season are calculated from the residuals $(Y - T)$ to represent the seasonal variation.

14.2.2.3   CYCLICAL COMPONENT

The cyclical components can be determined by the method of moving averages to the residuals $(Y - T - S)$.

14.2.2.4   RANDOM FLUCTUATIONS

The random fluctuations are obtained by subtracting the trend, seasonal variation, and cyclical component from the data. That is, it is obtained by

$$R = (Y - T - S - C)$$

14.2.2.5   NUMERICAL DEMONSTRATION

The following table shows the bimonthly number of out-patients registrations of dissociation disorder patients over a period of five years at a general hospital psychiatric unit.

Year	January–February	March–April	May–June	July–August	September–October	November–December	Total
1996	5	7	3	5	3	6	29
1997	1	6	7	4	3	5	26
1998	2	4	6	2	4	2	20
1999	4	7	7	5	5	5	33
2000	2	9	6	10	7	2	36
Total	14	33	29	26	22	20	144

A scanning of the figures in the last column of the table concludes an upward trend of the series. The series gradually decrease up to the year

1998 and increase thereafter. The figures in the last row of the table indicate a seasonal peak during March–April. In determining the trend, x is taken from 1 (January–February 1996) to 30 (November–December 2000). It may be computed that

$$T = 3.9 + 0.06x$$

In decomposition of seasonal variation, the trend is subtracted from the observations (y) in order to get the sum of the seasonal variation, cyclical component, and random fluctuations as shown in the table. The resultants (sum of seasonal variation, cyclical variation, and random fluctuations) are as shown below:

Year	January–February	March–April	May–June	July–August	September–October	November–December
1996	1.0	2.9	−1.1	0.8	−1.2	1.7
1997	−3.3	1.6	2.6	−0.5	−1.6	0.4
1998	−2.7	−0.7	1.2	−2.8	−0.9	−3.0
1999	−1.0	2.0	1.9	−0.2	−0.2	−0.3
2000	−3.3	3.6	0.6	4.5	1.5	−3.1
Mean (seasonal)	−1.9	1.9	1.0	0.4	−0.5	−0.9

The last row of the table indicates the seasonal variation. The seasonal variation is subtracted from the data in the last table in order to obtain the sum of the cyclical variation and random fluctuations as shown below:

Year	January–February	March–April	May–June	July–August	September–Oct	November–December	Mean (cyclical)
1996	2.9	1.1	−2.2	0.5	−0.7	2.7	0
1997	−1.5	−0.3	1.5	−0.9	−1.1	1.3	−0.2
1998	−0.8	−2.6	0.2	−3.2	−0.4	−2.0	−1.5
1999	0.9	0.1	0.9	−0.5	0.3	0.7	0.4
2000	−1.5	1.7	−0.5	4.2	2.0	−2.7	0.6

The last column of the table indicates the cyclical component.

The graphical representation of the trend, seasonal variation, and the cyclical components are shown in the following Figure 14.1.

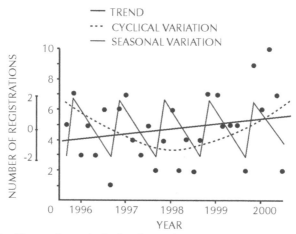

FIGURE 14.1   Time series analysis showing various components.

KEYWORDS

- **Cyclical component**
- **Seasonal variation**
- **Time series analysis**

CHAPTER 15

MULTIVARIATE STATISTICAL METHODS

CONTENTS

15.1   PROFILE TECHNIQUES

15.1.1   THREE-VARIABLES PROFILE

The profile techniques simultaneously plot data on several variables. Thus, a profile is best described as histogram on each variable, connecting between variables by identifying cases. The various objectives of profile techniques make it difficult to give complete explicit instructions for constructing profiles. It is especially useful in informally suggesting possible clusters of similar cases and also groups of similar variables.

Example: Let the percentage frequencies of male gender, percentage frequencies of high-income group, and percentage frequencies of admitted patients of five diagnostic categories of 409 psychiatric patients registered at NIMHANS hospital are as shown in the following table.

Variable	Organic psychosis (14)	Substance use disorders (58)	Schizophrenia (124)	Affective disorders (139)	Neurotic disorders (74)
1. Male (%)	79	98	53	53	45
2. High income (%)	21	31	36	44	53
3. Rate of admission (%)	43	71	40	30	11

The initial analysis consists of single-variable summaries such as minimum and maximum percentages. The profile diagram is drawn as shown in Figure 15.1.

It can be grasped that the variable male gender and rate of admission are similar. Further, it may be grasped that schizophrenia and affective disorders are similar with respect to these three variables.

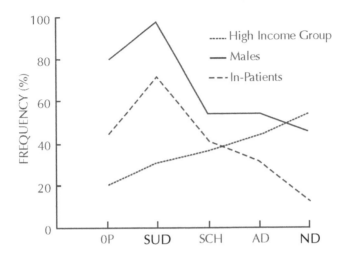

FIGURE 15.1   Profile showing percentage frequencies of diagnostic categories on three variables.

15.2   MULTIVARIATE CORRELATION COEFFICIENTS

15.2.1   *PARTIAL CORRELATION COEFFICIENT*

The correlation coefficient between two variables after eliminating the effect of the other variables is called partial correlation coefficient.

Example: The partial correlation coefficient between the fathers' heights and the sons' heights after eliminating the influence of mothers' heights. The partial correlation coefficient between the two variables (denoted by 1 and 2) after eliminating the influence of the third variable (denoted by 3) is given by

$$r_{12.3} = \frac{r_{12} - r_{13}r_{23}}{\sqrt{\left(1 - r_{13}^2\right)\left(1 - r_{23}^2\right)}}$$

The partial correlation coefficient lies between -1 and 1.

15.2.2 MULTIPLE CORRELATION COEFFICIENT

In multivariate data, the correlation between one variable and the combined influence of the other variables is known as multiple correlation coefficients. In trivariate data (three variables data), it is given by

$$R^2_{1(23)} = \frac{r_{12}^2 + r_{13}^2 - 2r_{12}r_{13}r_{23}}{(1 - r_{23}^2)}$$

The multiple correlation coefficient lies between 0 and 1.

Example: Let us assume the marks scored by 5 students in mathematics (denoted by variable 1), statistics (denoted by variable 2), and psychology (denoted by variable 3) as given below:

Student	Variable 1	Variable 2	Variable 3
1	4	7	10
2	2	4	7
3	3	1	8
4	0	3	6
5	6	5	4

For this data, the correlation coefficient matrix is computed and presented below:

	Variable 1	Variable 2	Variable 3
Variable 1	-	0.45	−0.15
Variable 2	-	-	0.20
Variable 3	-	-	-

For this data, the partial correlation coefficient between mathematics (variable 1) and statistics (variable 2) after eliminating the influence of psychology (variable 3) is calculated as follows:

$$r_{12.3} = \frac{0.45 - (-0.15)(0.20)}{\sqrt{(1-(-0.15^2))(1-0.20^2)}} = \frac{0.45 + 0.03}{\sqrt{(1-0.0225)(1-0.04)}} = 0.4955$$

For this data, the multiple correlation coefficient between mathematics (variable 1) and the combined influence of statistics (variable 2) and psychology (variable 3) are calculated as follows:

$$R^2_{1(23)} = \frac{0.45^2 + 0.20^2 - 2 \times 045 \times 0.20(-0.15)}{1-(-0.15)^2} = \frac{0.2025 + 0.04 + 0.027}{(1-0.0225)} = \frac{0.2695}{0.9775} = 0.2757$$

Hence,

$$R_{1(23)} = 0.525$$

15.3   MULTIPLE REGRESSION ANALYSIS

In multiple regression analysis, we have more than one independent variables $(x_1, x_2, \ldots x_k)$. The multiple regression analysis is based on the assumption that all the variables are normally distributed. A regression of k independent variables upon a dependent variable may be expressed as follows:

$$y = a + b_1 x_1 + b_2 x_2 + \ldots + b_k x_k$$

where a is a constant term

b_i are the simple partial regression coefficients

15.3.1   TWO-INDEPENDENT VARIABLES REGRESSION ANALYSIS

In case of two-independent variables (x_1 and x_2), we have the regression equation as given below:

$$y = a + b_1 x_1 + b_2 x_2$$

where

$$a = \bar{y} - b_1 \bar{x}_1 - b_2 \bar{x}_2$$

$$b_1 = \frac{(\sum X_1 Y)(\sum X_2^2) - (\sum X_2 Y)(\sum X_1 X_2)}{(\sum X_1^2)(\sum X_2^2) - (\sum X_1 X_2)^2}$$

$$b_2 = \frac{(\sum X_2 Y)(\sum X_1^2) - (\sum X_1 Y)(\sum X_1 X_2)}{(\sum X_1^2)(\sum X_2^2) - (\sum X_1 X_2)^2}$$

$$X_1 = (x_1 - \bar{x}_1)$$

$$X_2 = (x_2 - \bar{x}_2)$$

$$Y = (y - \bar{y})$$

Example: Let us assume that we have data of five students on two independent variables (IQ and personality scores) and dependent variable (success scores) as shown below:

Student	I Q (x_1)	Personality score (x_2)	Success score (y)
1	91	4	7
2	100	2	4
3	109	3	1
4	97	0	3
5	103	6	5
Mean	100	3	4

Computation table

Student	x_1	x_2	y	X_1	X_2	Y	X_1^2	X_2^2	$X_1 X_2$	$X_1 Y$	$X_2 Y$
1	91	4	7	−9	1	3	81	1	−9	−27	3
2	100	2	4	0	−1	0	0	1	0	0	0
3	109	3	1	9	0	−3	81	0	0	−27	0
4	97	0	3	−3	−3	−1	9	9	9	3	3
5	103	6	5	3	3	1	9	9	9	3	3
Total	500	15	20	0	0	0	180	20	9	−48	9

$$b_1 = \frac{(-48)(20) - (9 \times 9)}{(180 \times 20) - 9} = \frac{-10.41}{3591} = -0.290$$

$$b_2 = \frac{9 \times 180 - (-48)9}{(180 \times 20) - 9} = \frac{2052}{3591} = 0.5714$$

$a = 4 - (-0.29) \times 100 - (0.5714) \times 3 = 4 + 29 - 1.7142 = 31.2858$

$\hat{y} = 31.2858 - 0.29x_1 + 0.5714 x_2$

That is, success score $= 31.2858 - 0.29$ IQ $+ 0.5714$ personality score

Now, the predicted values of the dependent variable ($\hat{y}$) are computed as shown in the following table:

Student	y	$\hat{y}$	$(y-\hat{y})$
1	7	7.25	−0.25
2	4	3.42	0.58
3	1	1.33	−0.33
4	3	3.15	−0.15
5	5	4.85	0.15
Total	20	20.00	0

The estimates are fairly close to the actual values and the correlation between the two is 0.996, which is the multiple correlation coefficient denoted by R. This is the maximum possible correlation between the dependent variable and any linear combination of the independent variables.

15.4 MULTIVARIATE ANALYSIS OF VARIANCE

15.4.1 TWO-GROUPS AND TWO VARIABLES

15.4.1.1 LAYOUT

The layout of multivariate analysis of variance (MANOVA) is as given in the example.

15.4.1.2   HYPOTHESES

The means of a sample on several variables may be thought of a single point in a space that has as many dimensions as there are variables. The MANOVA technique may be employed to test the significance of the difference between multivariate means of several groups.

15.4.1.3   TEST STATISTIC

The chi-square test statistic is given by

$$\chi^2 = - \left(\sum n_g \right) l_n \text{ with df} = (g-1)\, t$$

where g is the number of groups
  t is the number of variables (tests)

$$L = \frac{W}{T}$$

where W is the pooled within group sum of squares and sum of products matrix
  T is the total sum of squares and cross-products
  The L-criterion lies between 0 and 1. If $L = 0$, then there is no between groups variances or covariances. This means that every group has the same mean score on a particular variable and that this is true for all the variables.
  Example: Let us suppose that the marks scored by three arts graduates and the marks scored by three science graduates on two aptitude tests are given below:

Arts graduate	Test 1	Test 2
Graduate 1	3	6
Graduate 2	4	4
Graduate 3	5	8
Mean	4	6

Science graduate	Test 1	Test 2
Graduate 4	1	2
Graduate 5	2	0
Graduate 6	3	4
Mean	2	2

For this data, we calculated the sum of squares and sum of products matrix of each diagnostic groups.

$$W = W_1 + W_2$$

$$W_1 = \begin{bmatrix} 2 & 2 \\ 2 & 8 \end{bmatrix} \quad W_2 = \begin{bmatrix} 2 & 2 \\ 2 & 8 \end{bmatrix} \quad W = \begin{bmatrix} 4 & 4 \\ 4 & 16 \end{bmatrix}$$

$$T = T_1 + T_2$$

$$T_1 = \begin{bmatrix} 5 & 8 \\ 8 & 20 \end{bmatrix} \quad T_2 = \begin{bmatrix} 5 & 8 \\ 8 & 20 \end{bmatrix} \quad T = \begin{bmatrix} 10 & 16 \\ 16 & 40 \end{bmatrix}$$

$$L = \frac{W}{T} = \frac{(64-16)}{(400-256)} = \frac{48}{144} = \frac{1}{3}$$

Hence,

$\chi^2 = -6\, l_n(\frac{1}{3}) = -6\,(-1.0986\,) = 6.592$, with $df = (2-1)\,2 = 2$

Since the calculated value is more than the table value of $\chi^2(2) = 5.99$, we reject the null hypotheses ($P < 0.05$, significant). That is, we have the evidence that the two groups are drawn from populations that differ in their mean quantities of x or in their mean quantities of y or in some compound of the two.

15.5   ANALYSIS OF MULTI-DIMENSIONAL CONTINGENCY TABLES

All the tables that simultaneously present data of more than two qualitative variables are known as multi-dimensional contingency table. A three-dimensional $r \times c \times l$ contingency table has r rows, c columns, and l layer categories. The observed frequency in the ijk-th cell of the table is denoted by $O_{ijk}(i = 1, 2, \dots r; j = 1, 2, \dots c; k = 1, 2, \dots l)$. By summing the O_{ijk} over different subscripts, various marginal totals may be obtained.

15.5.1 ANALYSIS OF THREE-DIMENSIONAL CONTINGENCY TABLE

2 × 2 × 2 contingency table

		Variable k			
	Category 1		Category 2		
Variable *j*	Category 1	Category 2	Category 1	Category 2	Total
Variable i Category 1	O_{111}	O_{121}	O_{112}	O_{122}	$O_{1..}$
Category 2	O_{211}	O_{221}	O_{212}	O_{222}	$O_{2..}$
Total	$O_{.11}$	$O_{.21}$	$O_{.12}$	$O_{.22}$	
Total		$O_{..1}$		$O_{..2}$	Total

15.5.1.1 HYPOTHESES

The null hypotheses state that the three variables are mutually independent. That is,

$$H_0 : P_{ijk} = P_{i..} P_{.j.} P_{..k}$$

where P_{ijk} represents the probability of an observation occurring in the ijk-th cell, and $P_i P_j P_k$ are the marginal probabilities of the row, column, and layer variables, respectively. When H_0 is true, the expected values are obtained as follows:

$$e_{ilk} = \frac{Oi.. \ O.j. \ O..k}{n^2}$$

15.5.1.2   TEST STATISTIC

It is given by

$$\chi^2 = \sum\sum\sum \frac{(O_{ijk} - e_{ijk})^2}{e_{ijk}} \quad df = rcl - r - c - l + 2$$

Example: The following table shows data concerning classroom behavior of 97 school children. Three variables are involved in the table. The first variable is a teacher's rating of classroom behavior classified into non-deviant and deviant. The second variable is the home risk index based on several items such as overcrowding thought to be related to deviant behavior. The third variable is an index of the adversity of school conditions based on items such as pupil turnover.

		Adversity of school conditions (k):				Total
		Low		High		
Home risk index (*j*):		NAR	AR	NAR	AR	Total
Classroom Non-deviant		16	7	20	37	80
Behavior(i):						
	Deviant	1	1	4	11	17
	Total	17	8	24	48	97
	Total		25		72	97

NAR, not at risk and AR, at risk.

We have computed the expected values as shown in the following example:

$$e_{111} = \frac{80 \times 41 \times 25}{97 \times 97} = 8.72$$

The full set of expected values is given below in the following table:

		Adversity of school conditions (k):				Total
		Low		High		
Home risk index (j):		NAR	AR	NAR	AR	Total
Classroom Behavior (i):	Non-deviant	8.72	11.90	25.10	34.28	80
	Deviant	1.85	2.53	5.33	7.28	17
Total		10.57	14.43	30.43	41.56	97

$\chi^2 = 12.905$ df $= 4$, $P < 0.05$, significant.

KEYWORDS

- **Correlation coefficient**
- **MANCOVA**

CHAPTER 16

CLUSTER ANALYSIS

CONTENTS

16.1   FUNCTIONS OF CLUSTER ANALYSIS

16.1.1   CLASSIFICATION

Researchers in all fields need to make and revise classifications continuously. For example, researchers in psychiatric field need to make classification of mental patients based on psychiatric test scores in order to improve their understanding of mental illness and plan for its treatments. The proportional incidence of one symptom or another indicates whether it is a characteristic feature of the disease or not. The identification of signs and symptoms of a disorder or syndrome is the major concern of psychiatrists. Inadequate parental control of hyperactivity children is found by chance, and it is found in almost every case of conduct disorder children.

16.1.2   SHEDDING LIGHT ON THE PREVIOUSLY MADE HYPOTHESES

The cluster analysis may be useful in shedding light on the previously made hypotheses. For example, there has long been controversy over the classification of depressed patients. The issues involved here have been reviewed on a number of occasions. Several attempts have been made to establish the validity of classifying such patients into reactive and endogenous groups. The problem has been tackled with some success by using cluster analysis techniques.

16.1.3   PREDICTION

The cluster analysis may be useful to produce groups that form the basis of a classification scheme useful in latter studies for predictive purpose of some kind. For example, a cluster analysis applied to data consisting of a sample of psychiatric patients may produce groups of patients who react differently when treated with some drug. Thus, it enables us to decide whether a drug is suitable for a particular type of patients. Such a procedure was used in an investigation of the useful of amitriptyline in the treatment of depression.

16.1.4   EVALUATION OF PROGRAMS

The cluster analysis is useful as multivariate evaluation of programs.

16.1.5   FURTHER FUNCTIONS

The other functions of cluster analysis include the following:
  (a) Exploring the data and generate hypotheses
  (b) Summarizing the data and display
  (c) Naming the resultant groups and giving explanations
  (d) Fitting models

16.2   HIERARCHICAL CLUSTER ANALYSIS

In hierarchical clustering methods, the clusters are classified into groups, and the process is repeated at different levels to form a tree. There are two types of hierarchical methods: divisive techniques and agglomerative techniques.

16.2.1   HIERARCHICAL DIVISIVE CLUSTER ANALYSIS

The divisive clustering methods partition the set of entities successfully into finer partitions. Thus, the divisive techniques will finally split the entire set of data into groups each containing a single entity.

16.2.2   HIERARCHICAL AGGLOMERATIVE CLUSTER ANALYSIS

The hierarchical agglomerative clustering methods proceed by a series of successive fusions of n entities into groups. Thus, the agglomerative techniques ultimately reduce the data to a single cluster containing all the entities.

16.2.3   DENDROGRAM

The results of both agglomerative techniques and divisive techniques may be presented in the form of a dendrogram. A dendrogram is a two-dimensional diagram that illustrates the fusions or partitions that have been made at each successive level.

16.3   MEASURES OF SIMILARITY AND DISSIMILARITY BETWEEN PERSONS

16.3.1   MEASURES OF SIMILARITY

The similarity measure (association coefficients) between two individuals (patients) are usually calculated for binary data (presence or absence) of a variable in an individual or polychotomous data (present or absent of a category of polychotomous variable). The primary step in the calculation of the coefficients is to arrange the data in a 2×2 matching table as shown below:

2×2 matching table

		Individual *j*	
		Present	**Absent**
Individual *i*	Present	a	b
	Absent	c	d

Many different coefficients have been suggested for this data.

16.3.1.1   SIMPLE MATCHING COEFFICIENT

The simple matching coefficient between two individuals *i* and *j* is given by

$$SMC_{ij} = \frac{(a+d)}{(a+b+c+d)}$$

16.3.1.2   JACCARD'S COEFFICIENT

The Jaccard's coefficient between two individuals i and j is given by

$$JC_{ij} = \frac{a}{(a+b+C)}$$

16.3.2   MEASURES OF DISSIMILARITY

The dissimilarity measures (distance measures) are usually calculated for counting data (frequency data) and continuous data.

16.3.2.1   SQUARED EUCLIDIAN DISTANCE

The squared Euclidian distance between two individuals (patients) i and j is given by,

$$SED_{ij} = \Sigma \left(x_{ik} - x_{jk} \right)^2$$

where x_{ik} is the value of ith individual on the kth variable.

16.3.2.2   ABSOLUTE EUCLIDIAN DISTANCE

The absolute Euclidian distance between two individuals (patients) i and j is given by

$$AED_{ij} = \Sigma \left| x_{ik} - x_{jk} \right|$$

16.3.3   CHOICE OF VARIABLES AND STANDARDIZATION

The choice of variables to be included is an important issue in clustering analysis. Ideally, variables should be chosen within the context of an explicitly stated theory that is used to support the classification. If the data are not of the same scale values, they are commonly standardized to a mean of zero and to unit variance.

16.4   HIERARCHICAL AGGLOMERATIVE CLUSTERING METHODS

The basic procedure with all agglomerative methods is similar. They begin with the computation of a matrix of proximity (similarity or dissimilarity) between the entities. At any particular stage, the techniques fuse individuals or groups of individuals that are closest. Each fusion decreases the number of groups by 1. Differences between hierarchical agglomerative methods arise because of the different ways of defining proximity between groups (clusters).

16.4.1   SINGLE-LINKAGE METHOD

In single-linkage method (nearest neighbor method), the distance between groups is defined as the distance between their closest members. That is,

$$d_{i(jk)} = \text{minimum } (d_{ij}, d_{ik})$$

where the single-linkage method can be used with both similarity and distance measures. The major drawback of this method is that it has the tendency to form long and elongated clusters.

16.4.2   COMPLETE LINKAGE METHOD

In the complete linkage method (furthest neighbor method), the distance between groups is defined as the distance between their most remote pair of individuals. That is,

$$d_{i(jk)} = \text{maximum } (d_{ij}, d_{ik})$$

This method has a tendency to find relatively compact and hyper spherical clusters composed of highly similar cases.

16.4.3   *AVERAGE LINKAGE BETWEEN MERGED GROUPS*

In the average linkage between the merged groups, the distance between the two groups is defined as the average of the distances of all pair-wise combinations between the individuals in the two groups. That is,

$$d_{i(jk)} = \text{mean} \ (d_{ij}, \ d_{ik})$$

In this method, a cluster is defined as a group of clusters in which each member has a greater mean similarity with a member of the same cluster than it does with all members of any other cluster.

16.4.4   *AVERAGE LINKAGE WITHIN THE NEW GROUP*

In the average linkage within the new group (within-groups linkage),the distance between two groups is defined as the average of the distances of all pair-wise combinations of all individuals in the two groups. That is,

$$d_{i(jk)} = \text{mean} \ (d_{ij}, \ d_{ik,} d_{jk})$$

This method frequently gives results that are a little different from those obtained with the complete linkage method.

16.4.5   *MINIMUM VARIANCE METHOD*

The minimum variance method (Ward's method) is designed to generate clusters in such a way that the variance within a cluster is minimum. The clusters found in this method can be ordered in terms of their overall elevation.

16.5   DETERMINATION OF NUMBER OF CLUSTERS

16.5.1   *EMPIRICAL INVESTIGATIONS*

Hierarchical cluster analysis gives configuration for every number of clusters from one up to the number of entities in the data. We usually want the clusters to be few in number and to be well defined. However, the purpose of the classification is also a factor. Ultimately, we want the classification to be judged valid. Thus, we want to get number of clusters that make it to work the best. Often it is expected that few well-defined clusters would work better than many clusters.

16.5.2 ANALYTICAL METHODS

Some researchers in psychiatry have been preoccupied with an idea of optimum number of clusters rather than considering the possibility of several alternative classifications, each reflecting different aspects of the data. There are several analytical methods to determine the number of clusters, which are based on the within- and between-cluster distances. Maximizing the between-cluster sum of squares is essentially the criterion used here.

16.6   PARTITIONING CLUSTER ANALYSIS

The partitioning clustering methods are designed to cluster data units into a single classification of k clusters, where k is determined as part of the hierarchical cluster analysis. The central idea in most of the these methods is to choose some initial partition of the data units and then alter cluster membership so as to obtain a better partition. Most of these methods use-distant procedures with respect to the method of initiating clusters and a method of locating some or all of the entities to other clusters once an initial classificatory process has been completed.

16.6.1 METHODS OF INITIATING CLUSTERS

These are two basic ways for initiating clusters: one is by using seed points and other by selecting an appropriate starting partition. The use of seed points approach consists in finding k-points (seed points) in the p-dimensional space, which acts as initial estimates of the cluster center. The seed points can be generated (1) by subjectively choosing any k data units from the data set and (2) by using the centroids of the k clusters of classification obtained by hierarchical methods. When seed points are used, entities are allocated to the seed points to those whose center they are nearest. The seed points may remain stationary throughout the assignment of the full data set.

16.6.2 METHODS FOR REALLOCATION OF ENTITIES

The methods for reallocating entities deal with the ways in which cases are reassigned to clusters. There are two basic types: the k-means passes and the hill-climbing passes. The k-means passes are also referred to as the nearest centroid sorting passes. This simply involves the reassignment of cases to the clusters with the nearest centroid. The k-means passes can be either combinatorial or non-combinatorial. The former method requires the calculation of the centroid of the cluster after each change in its membership, whereas the latter method recalculates the cluster centroid only after an entire pass through the data has been completed.

16.6.3 FORGY'S METHOD

Among the several methods suited to the basic problem of sorting the data units into a fixed number of clusters, the method suggested by Forgy is very commonly used. This method suggests a very simple algorithm consisting of the following sequence of steps:

Step1: Begin with any desired initial configuration. Go to step 2 if beginning with a set of seed points. Go to step 3 if beginning with a partition of the data units.

Step 2: Allocate each data units to the cluster with the nearest seed points. The seed points remain fixed for a few cycle through the entire data set.

Step 3: Compute new seed points as the centroids of the cluster of data units.

Step 4: Alternate steps 2 and 3 until the process converges. That is, continue until no data unit changes their cluster membership at step 2.

16.6.4 REDDY'S VARIANT METHOD

Step1: Subjectively choose k data units each from the clusters of classification obtained by hierarchical methods.

Step 2:Allocate each data units to the cluster with the nearest seed points. The seed points remain fixed for a few cycle through the entire data set.

Step 3: Compute new seed points as the centroids of the cluster of data units.

Step 4: Alternate steps 2 and 3 until the process converges. That is, continue until no data unit changes their cluster membership at Step 2.

16.7   VALIDATION OF RESULTANT CLUSTERS

Different clustering techniques can and do generate different solutions to the same data set, and hence a number of validation techniques have been developed to provide some relief to this problem. The strategy of cluster analysis is structure seeking although its operation is structure imposing, and therefore the key to use cluster analysis is to know when these groups are real and not merely imposed on the data by the method. Various intuitively reasonable procedures have been suggested for evaluating the stability and the usefulness of the set of clusters obtained.

16.7.1   METHOD OF REPLICATION

In method of replication, the same dataset may be cluster analyzed by different methods. The solution by the majority of the methods should be similar to say that the data are clearly structured.

16.7.2   TESTS OF SIGNIFICANCE OF INTERNAL VARIABLES

In tests of significance on variables used to create clusters, the clustering solution is validated by applying ANOVA/MANOVA or chi-square as tests of significance of the difference between clusters on these variables that are used to create clusters. Since these tests are positive regardless of whether clusters exist in the data or not, they must be performed on a controlled data set to draw valid conclusions on their distinguishability.

16.7.3   TESTS OF SIGNIFICANCE OF EXTERNAL VARIABLES

In tests of significance on external variables, the obtained clusters are compared on variables of interest, which were not included in the original analysis. If differences between clusters persist with respect to these variables, then there is some evidence that a useful solution has been obtained, in the sense that by stating that a particular entity belongs to a particular cluster, we convey information on variables not used to produce the clusters.

16.7.4   METHOD OF MARKER SAMPLE

In psychiatric research, especially in making diagnosis, the sample from major clinical diagnostic categories is pooled together as marker sample to aid in validating the cluster solution. An adequate solution should place dissimilar subjects into different clusters and provide some indication of the number of clusters required to provide reasonable differentiation. For example, it would have been conceptually inconsistent for a given cluster solution to classify numerous psychosomatic and psychotics together in the same cluster.

16.7.5   ASSOCIATION WITH PRE-PROGRAM ASSESSMENT TEST SCORES

In evaluation of programs, the resultant clusters are evaluated by tests of significance of association with preprogram assessment test scores.

16.7.6   NUMERICAL DEMONSTRATION

Let us suppose that we have scores of six patients on two diagnostic tests as shown below:

Patient	Test 1	Test 2
A	3	6
B	4	4
C	5	8
D	1	2
E	2	0
F	3	4

The squared Euclidian distance matrix is computed as shown below. For example, the squared Euclidian distance between A and B is given by

$$(3 - 4)^2 + (6 - 4)^2 = 1 + 4 = 5.$$

Patient	A	B	C	D	E	F
A	-	5	8	20	37	4
B	-	-	17	13	20	1
C	-	-	-	52	73	20
D	-	-	-	-	5	8
E	-	-	-	-	-	17
F	-	-	-	-	-	-

Let us select single-linkage method for the purpose of classification. As a first step in the application, patients B and F are fused to form a cluster (BF), since the distance between them is the smallest. The distance between the cluster (BF), and the remaining four patients are obtained as shown in the following distance matrix table.

Clusters	BF	A	C	D	E
BF	-	5	20	13	17
A	-	-	8	20	37
C	-	-	-	52	73
D	-	-	-	-	5
E	-	-	-	-	-

The smallest entry in the above-cited matrix is 5, which is the distance between patients D and E. Hence, they are fused to form the second cluster (DE). Now, the distance matrix is as given below:

Cluster	BF	A	C	DE
BF	-	5	17	20
A	-	-	8	37
C	-	-	-	73
DE	-	-	-	-

It can be noted that the distance between the Patient A and the cluster (BF) is the smallest. They are fused to form the cluster (BFA). Now, the distance matrix is given by

Cluster	BFA	C	DE
BFA	-	8	20
C	-	-	73
DE	-	-	-

It can be noted that the distance between the patient C and the cluster (BFA) is the smallest. They are fused to form the cluster (BFAC). Now, the distance matrix is as given below:

Cluster	BFAC	DE
BFAC	-	20
DE	-	-

Finally, the cluster (BFAC) and (DE) are fused at a distance of 20 units to form a single cluster consisting of all the six patients.

The dendrogram is shown in Figure 16.1.

FIGURE 16.1   Dendrogram of six patients based on scores on two diagnostic tests.

KEYWORDS

- **Cluster analysis**
- **Dendrogram**
- **Jaccard's coefficient**

CHAPTER 17

DISCRIMINANT ANALYSIS

CONTENTS

17.1   TWO-GROUP DISCRIMINANT ANALYSIS

Here, we are provided with two classes (groups) of persons, and t measurements have been made on each person.

17.1.1   VECTOR OF WEIGHTS

We aim at finding out the weighing vector that when applied to some newly observed and unclassified person will assign him to one or other of the classes with the smallest probability of error. The vector of weights (w) which provides the optimum assignment is given by the following relation:

$$w = V^{-1} d$$

where V is the weighted average of the variance–covariance matrix. It is given by the following relation:

$$V = \frac{W_1 + W_2}{(n_1 + n_2 - 2)}$$

where d is the vector of differences between the t-pairs of means of the two groups.

17.1.2   CUT-OFF SCORE FOR CLASSIFICATION

Generally, for classification purpose, the appropriate cut-off point score is the half-way mark between the means of the discriminant scores of the two groups.

17.1.3   PROBABILITY OF MISCLASSIFICATION

The probability of misclassification is given by the following relation:

$$P(\text{mc}) = 0.5 - P(0.5 D)$$

where D^2 is the generalized distance (Mahalanobis D^2) between two groups. It is the inner product of the vector of difference d and the vector of weights w. That is,

$$D^2 = d'w = d' V^{-1} d$$

It can be shown that the D^2 is the difference between the means of the two groups on discriminant function scores. In addition it can be shown that half of D is a unit normal deviate. Hence, it can be used to determine the probability of misclassification. If we look it up in a table of Z-distribution, we find the probability of an individual who really belongs to one group will be incorrectly assigned to the other group by the discriminant function analysis.

17.2   K-GROUP DISCRIMINANT ANALYSIS

The technique of the linear discriminate analysis developed for the two groups can be extended to the case of more than two groups.

17.2.1   WEIGHT OF UNCLASSIFIED PERSON IN VARIOUS GROUPS

The weight of the unclassified person (undiagnosed patient) in the ith group (diagnosis) is given by the following relation:

$$w_i = p'l_i - \tfrac{1}{2} m_i'l_i$$

where p is the column vector of scores of the unclassified person. The l_i is the vector of weights for the ith group. It is given by

$$l_i = V^{-1} m_i$$

m_i is the vector of means of the ith group

The procedure is to assign the person to the group for which he obtains the highest score.

17.2.2 NUMERICAL DEMONSTRATION

Let us suppose that a child psychiatrist has to take a decision whether conduct disorder or hyperkinetic diagnosis may be more suitable for a child registered at a child guidance clinic. The information on which the decision is based on is derived from the scores of three genuine conduct disorder children and three genuine hyperkinetic children as the basis for our advice. The children obtained the following scores on two diagnostic tests:

Conduct disorder child	Test 1	Test 2
C1	3	6
C2	4	4
C3	5	8
Mean	4	6

Hyperkinetic child	Test 1	Test 2
C4	1	2
C5	2	0
C6	3	4
Mean	2	2

We calculated the sum of squares and sum of products matrix of each diagnostic groups.

$$W_1 = \begin{bmatrix} 2 & 2 \\ 2 & 8 \end{bmatrix} W_2 = \begin{bmatrix} 2 & 2 \\ 2 & 8 \end{bmatrix} W = \begin{bmatrix} 4 & 4 \\ 4 & 16 \end{bmatrix}$$

The weighted average of the variance–covariance matrix is as given below:

$$V = \begin{bmatrix} 4 & 4 \\ 4 & 16 \end{bmatrix} \Big/ 4 = \begin{bmatrix} 1 & 1 \\ 1 & 4 \end{bmatrix}$$

And $V^{-1} = \begin{bmatrix} \dfrac{4}{3} & \dfrac{-1}{3} \\ \dfrac{-1}{3} & \dfrac{1}{3} \end{bmatrix}$ and $d = \begin{pmatrix} 2 \\ 4 \end{pmatrix}$

Hence, $w = \begin{pmatrix} \dfrac{4}{3} \\ \dfrac{2}{3} \end{pmatrix}$

Now, the discriminate scores of the six children are calculated as shown in the following table. For example, the discriminate scores of the first child are calculated as follows:

$$\left(\frac{4}{3} \times 3 \right) + \left(\frac{2}{3} \times 6 \right) = 8$$

Conduct disorder child	Discriminate score
C1	8.00
C2	8.00
C3	12.00
Mean	9.33

Hyperkinetic child	Discriminate score
C4	2.67
C5	2.67
C6	6.67
Mean	4.00

The half-way mark (cut-off score) is given by

$$(9.33 + 4.00)/2 = 6.67$$

Let we support that the scores of an undiagnosed child are given by 2 and 5 on test 1 and 2, respectively. The discriminate scores of this child is calculated as,

$$(2 \times 4/3) + (5 \times 2/3) = (8/3 + 10/3) = 6.00$$

Since, this value is less than the cut-off score of 6.67, the child is most appropriately diagnosed as hyperkinetic child.

The generalized distance (D^2) is calculated as follows:

$$D^2 = (2 \ \ 4) \begin{pmatrix} \dfrac{4}{3} \\ \dfrac{2}{3} \end{pmatrix}$$

$$= (8/3 + 8/3) = 16/3 = 5.33$$

D^2 can also be obtained as follows:

D^2 = (mean of the first group) − (mean of the second group)

$= 9.33 - 4.00 = 5.33$

$D = 2.31$

Now,

$P(\text{mc}) = 0.50 - P(0.5 \times 2.31) = 0.50 - P(1.155)$

$= 0.05 - 0.37 = 0.13$

Thus, the probability of misclassification is 13 percent that means that we may expect 87 percent of our assignments(diagnosis) to be correct.

KEYWORDS

- **Cut-off score**
- **Hyperkinetic children**

CHAPTER 18

FACTOR ANALYSIS

CONTENTS

18.1   BASIC ELEMENTS OF FACTOR ANALYSIS

18.1.1   FACTOR LOADINGS

It is a matrix representing the correlations between different combinations of variables and factors. Let the L_{ij} is the factor loading of the ith factor on the jth variable ($i = 1,2\ldots k$ and $j = 1, 2 \ldots k$). Since the factors happen to be linear combinations of variables, the coordinates of each variable is measured to obtain what are called factor loadings. Such factor loadings represent the correlation between the particular variable and the factor. The higher the factor loadings, the more likely it is that the factor is underlying that variable. Factor loadings help in identifying which variables are associated with the particular factor. There are a number of ways by which factor analysis is done.

18.1.2   EXTRACTION OF FACTORS AND ROTATION

In the process of extraction of factor loadings, the rotation helps in arriving at a suitable pattern of factor loadings by maximizing high correlation and minimizing low ones. A simple structure can be observed by looking at the factor loading of each factor. If the factor loading is high (as high as 1) on one factor and a very low factor loading (as low as 0) on the other, it is said to possess a simple structure. If there is no simple structure, then the n-dimensional space of the factors should be rotated by an angle such that the factor loadings are revised to have a simple structure that will ease the process of interpreting the factors. Rotation could be orthogonal or oblique. The orthogonal rotation should be used under the assumption that the underlying factors are uncorrelated with each other. The "varimax" method is the commonly used orthogonal rotation technique.

18.1.3   EIGENVALUES OF FACTORS

It is the sum of squares of the factor loadings of all the variables on a factor. The eigenvalue of the ith factor is given by

$$EV_i = \sum L_{ij}^2$$

Thus, the eigenvalues are the measure of amount of total variance in the data explained by a factor. Factor analysis initially considers the number of factors to be same as the total number of variables. Looking at the eigenvalue, one can determine if the factor explains sufficient amount of variance to be considered as a meaningful factor.

18.1.3.1   SCREE PLOT

An eigen value of less than 1 essentially means that the factor explains less variance than a single variable, and therefore should not be considered to be a meaningful factor. The scree plot is a graphical presentation of eigenvalues of all of the factors initially considered for extraction. It is used to decide on the number of factors to be considered.

18.1.4   COMMUNALITIES OF VARIABLES

It is the sum of squares of the factor loadings of the *j*th variable on all factors. Thus, it is given by

$$\text{COM}_j = \Sigma \ L_{ij}^2$$

The communalities give the variance accounted for a particular variable by all the factors. Mathematically, it is the sum of squared loadings for a variable across all the factors. The higher the value of the communality for a particular variable after extraction, the higher the amount of variance explained by factors extracted.

18.1.5   FACTOR SCORES OF PERSONS

The factor scores are obtained for each person. With factor scores, one can also perform several other multivariate statistical methods such as cluster analysis, discriminate analysis, and multi-dimensional scaling.

18.2 PRINCIPAL COMPONENTS ANALYSIS

The principal components analysis (PCA) is a variant of factor analysis; both are data analysis techniques. In PCA, all the variance in the observed variable in analyzed; whereas in other factor analysis, only shared variance is analyzed. The PCA extracts the maximum sum of squares of the loadings for each factor in turn. Accordingly, the PCA explains more variance than the loadings obtained from any other method of factoring. It is assumed that all the variables are standardized. The aim of this method is to construct new variables (P_i) called principal components that are linear combinations of a given set of variables $x_j (j = 1 \dots k)$.

$$P_1 = L_{11}x_1 + L_{12}x_2 + \dots + L_{1k}x_k$$

$$P_2 = L_{21}x_1 + L_{22}x_2 + \dots + L_{2k}x_k$$

$$P_k = L_{k1}x_1 + L_{k2}x_2 + \dots + L_{kk}x_k$$

The L_{ij} are called loadings and are worked out in such a way that the extracted principal components satisfy two conditions. First, the principal components are uncorrelated (orthogonal). Second, the first principal component has the maximum variance, the second principal component has the next maximum, and so on.

18.2.1 NUMERICAL DEMONSTRATION

The centroid method of extraction of factors is a popular technique for factor analysis because of its ease in understanding and relatively simpler calculations in comparison with other techniques. The steps involved in extracting factors using this method are explained with an example. A researcher is interested in obtaining the set of disciplines that a student exhibit while taking up a test. The scores obtained in mathematics, statistics, and in psychology are as given in the following table.

Student	Mathematics (x_1)	Statistics (x_2)	Psychology (x_3)
1	6	6	2
2	4	4	1
3	4	1	2
4	1	2	3

Student	Mathematics (x_1)	Statistics (x_2)	Psychology (x_3)
5	4	3	3
6	4	4	3
7	3	3	3
8	7	7	2
9	5	3	2
10	5	4	1

The researcher has decided to break down the data into two factors, so that the data set that has three variables can be represented by two factors.

18.2.1.1   EXTRACTION OF FIRST FACTOR

We begin with calculating the correlation coefficients matrix as shown in Table 18.1(a).

TABLE 18.1 (a)   Correlation coefficient matrix (R_1)

	(x_1)	(x_2)	(x_3)
x_1	1.000	0.765	−0.482
x_2	0.765	1.000	−0.271
x_3	−0.482	−0.271	1.000

Next, we check that if the correlation matrix is positive manifold. This implies that all the values of the matrix are positive. If they are not, then we have to reflect variables that have negative values. Reflection is done by assigning a weight of −1 to variables having negative values and +1 to variables having positive values. We start with looking at the values column wise. The reflected matrix is shown in Table 18.1(b).

TABLE18.1 (b) Correlation coefficient matrix R'_1 with reflection on variable 3

	(x_1)	(x_2)	(x_3)	-
x_1	1.000	0.765	0.482	-
x_2	0.765	1.000	0.271	-
x_3	0.482	0.271	1.000	-
Sum (S_j)	2.247	2.036	1.753	6.036

Next, we calculate the first centroid factor. The sum (S_j) of each column of the matrix R'_1 is shown in the table.

$$\sqrt{T} = \sqrt{6.036} = 2.457$$

The calculations to determine the loading of factor 1 (L_{1j}) are summarized in Table18.1(c).

TABLE 18.1 (c) Calculations to determine the loading values of the factor 1 (L_{1j})

Variable (j)	S_j	F'_1	F_1
1	2.247	0.915	0.915
2	2.036	0.829	0.829
3	1.753	0.714	−0.714

$$F'_1 = \frac{S}{\sqrt{T}} = \frac{S}{2.457}$$

18.2.1.2 EXTRACTION OF SECOND FACTOR

Next, we calculate the second centroid factor. This is done by calculating a cross-product matrix that consists of the product of each pair of coefficients loadings L_{1j} as shown in Table18.2(a).

TABLE 18.2 (a)   Cross-product matrix

	0.915	**0.829**	**−0.714**
0.915	0.837	0.759	−0.653
0.829	0.759	0.687	−0.592
−0.714	−0.653	−0.592	0.510

The residual matrix R_2 is obtained by subtracting the cross-product matrix from R_1, and it is shown in Table18.2(b).

TABLE 18.2 (b)   Residual matrix R_2

	x_1	x_2	x_3	
	0.163	0.006	0.171	
	0.006	0.313	0.321	
	0.171	0.321	0.490	
Sum (S_j)	0.340	0.640	0.982	1.962

$$\sqrt{T} = \sqrt{1.962} = 1.401$$

From this table, it is clear that no variable have to be reflected. The second centroid factor loading L_{2j} are summarized in Table18.2(c), after multiplying with respective column weights.

TABLE 18.2 (c)   Calculations to determine loadings of factor 2 (L_{2j})

J	S_j	F'_2	F_2
1	0.340	0.243	0.243
2	0.640	0.457	0.457
3	0.982	0.701	0.701

$$F'_2 = \frac{S}{\sqrt{T}} = \frac{S}{1.401}$$

18.2.1.3   EXTRACTION OF THIRD FACTOR

Next, we calculate the third centroid factor. This is done by calculating a cross-product matrix that consists of the product of each pair of coefficients of loadings L_{2j}, as shown in Table18.3(a).

TABLE 18.3 (a)   Cross-product matrix

	0.243	0.457	0.701
0.243	0.059	0.111	0.170
0.457	0.111	0.209	0.320
0.701	0.170	0.320	0.491

The residual matrix R_3 is obtained by subtracting the cross-product matrix from R_2, and it is shown in Table18.3(b).

TABLE 18.3 (b)   Residual matrix R_3

	x_1	x_2	x_3
x_1	0.104	−0.105	0.001
x_2	−0.105	0.104	0.001
x_3	0.001	0.001	−0.001

Residual matrix R'_3 with reflections on variables 1, 2, and 3 is given in Table 18.3(c)

TABLE 18.3 (c)   Residual matrix R'_3 with reflections on variables 1, 2, and 3

	x_1	x_2	x_3	-
x_1	0.104	0.105	0.001	-
x_2	0.105	0.104	0.001	-
x_3	0.001	0.001	0.001	-
Sum (S_j)	0.210	0.210	0.003	0.423

$$\sqrt{T} = \sqrt{0.423} = 0.650$$

The third centroid factor loadings are summarized in Table18.3(d) after multiplying with the respective column weights.

TABLE 18.3 (d)   Calculation to determine loadings of factor3 (L_{3j})

J	S_j	F'_3	F_3
1	0.210	0.323	−0.323
2	0.210	0.323	−0.323
3	0.003	0.005	−0.005

$$F'_3 = \frac{S}{\sqrt{T}} = \frac{S}{0.650}$$

18.2.1.4   ANALYSIS OF THE RESULTS

Loadings of the three factors on three variables is given in Table 18.4

TABLE 18.4   Loadings of the three factors

Variable	Factor 1	Factor 2	Factor 3	Communality (COM$_j$)
x_1	0.915	0.243	−0.323	1.000
x_2	0.829	0.457	−0.323	1.000
x_3	−0.714	0.701	−0.005	1.000
Eigenvalues (EV$_j$)	2.034	0.759	0.209	3.002
Proportion of total variance	0.678	0.253	0.069	1.000
Cumulative proportion of common variance	0.678	0.931	1.000	-

Next, we assign each variable to the factor with which it has the maximum absolute loadings as shown in table. The rule for assignment of a variable to a particular factor is simple. We assign that variable to a factor that has its factor loading greater than 0.6. Therefore, looking at Table 18.4, we can say that variables and   load at factor1 as their individual loadings are greater than 0.6. The final assignment of variables to factors is summarized in Table 18.5.

TABLE 18.5   Assignment of variables to factors

Factor number	Name of the factor	Variables	Description
1	Mathematics discipline	x_1	Mathematics, statistics
		x_2	
2	Applied discipline	x_3	Psychology
3	-	-	-

The variables of mathematics and statistics can be replaced by a suitable factor that can be termed as mathematical discipline factor. Psychology subject form a factor called applied factor. About 68 percent of the total variance explained is due to factor 1, followed by factor 2 that explains another 25 percent. Cumulatively, factor 1 and 2 explains 93 percent of the total variance, and hence we could have considered these two factors and drop the third factor.

KEYWORDS

- **Centroid factor**
- **Communality**
- **Correlation coefficients**
- **Eigenvalue**
- **Factor analysis**
- **Varimax**

CHAPTER 19

META-ANALYSIS

CONTENTS

19.1   LOCATION AND SELECTION OF STUDIES FOR META-ANALYSIS

19.1.1   LOCATION OF STUDIES

19.1.1.1   PUBLICATION BIAS

The source of search for literature in meta-analysis includes the published literature, unpublished literature, uncompleted research reports and work in progress. Reliance on only published reports leads to publication bias- the bias resulting from the tendency to publish results that are statistically significant. Hence, the meta-analysis needs to obtain information from unpublished research also. Contact with colleagues, experts in the applied field, and other informed channels can be important sources of information on published, uncompleted, and ongoing studies.

19.1.2   SELECTION OF STUDIES

Given a vast quantity of heterogeneous literature, suitable studies have to be selected for a meta-analysis. The inclusion and exclusion criteria relate to quality and to the combinability of patients and out-come.

19.2   END-POINTS OF PRIMARY STUDIES

Meta-analysis is a two-stage process. In the first stage, the end-points (summary statistics) are collected from each primary study.

19.2.1   A LIST OF END-POINTS

The important end-points are the following:
1. Uncontrolled studies: Proportion/percentage, mean response, etc.
2. Controlled studies: Risk difference, risk ratio, odds ratio, mean difference, standardized mean difference, etc.
3. Critical ratios: Z values, χ^2 values, t-values, F-ratios, etc.
4. Effects sizes: Glass C, Hedges g, Cohen's d, etc.

19.2.1.1 COHEN'S d

It is given by

$$d = \frac{(\overline{x}_1 - \overline{x}_2)}{s}$$

where $\overline{x}_1$ is the mean of the first group
$\overline{x}_2$ is the mean of the second group
s is the pooled estimate of the standard deviations of the two groups
where s is given by

$$s = \sqrt{\frac{(n_1 - 1)S_1^2 + (n_2 - 1)S_2^2}{(n_1 + n_2 - 2)}}$$

19.2.2 TRANSFORMATION OF END-POINTS

All the studies selected for a meta-analysis may provide different end-points (data-points). In such cases, a transformation to common end-points is necessary. It is convenient to transform different statistics to the correlation coefficient 'r' before proceeding with further analysis. Below is a list of important transformations. When the end-point is

Contingency Coefficient, $\quad r = CC$

Phi-coefficient, $\quad r = \emptyset$

Z-value, $\quad r = \dfrac{Z}{\sqrt{n}}$

t-value, $\quad r = \dfrac{t}{\sqrt{t^2 + df}}$

F-value, $\quad r = \dfrac{SS_B}{SS_T}$

Cohen's d, $\quad r = \sqrt{\dfrac{d^2}{d^2 + 4}}$

19.3   QUALITY ASSESSMENT OF SELECTED STUDIES

Methods of quality assessment provide a systematic approach to describe primary studies and explain heterogeneity. A formal approach to decide the ultimate inclusion status of a study may be undertaken by using a penal of judges/experts.

19.3.1   A LIST OF QUALITY ASSESSMENT ITEMS

The important quality assessment items include the following:
1. The report: principal author, year of publication, source/journal, etc.
2. The study: scope, population, etc.
3. The patients: age, sex, socio-economic status, etc.
4. Study design: observational/experimental, random sampling/randomization, non-response error/attrition rate, etc.
5. Treatment: dose and timings, duration, mode of delivery, etc.
6. Effect size: effect size, sample size, nature of outcome, etc.

19.3.2   INTERNAL VALIDITY AND EXTERNAL VALIDITY

The internal validity of a study is the extent to which systematic error (bias) is minimized. Such biases are the selection bias, performance bias, detection bias, and attrition bias. The external validity is the extent to which the results of the study provide a correct basis for applicability to other circumstances. Thus, the internal validity is a prerequisite for external validity.

19.4   META-ANALYSIS MASTER SHEET

The first step in meta-analysis is to prepare a master sheet (data point-stable). The first column in the master sheet consists of the list of selected studies according to their chronological order of publications.

19.4.1   STATISTICAL HETEROGENEITY AND CLINICAL HETEROGENEITY

The last column of the table consists of their respective end-points or their transformed values in order to notice the statistical heterogeneity. The information on relevant variables (quality assessment items) isentered in the master sheet in order to notice the clinical heterogeneity.

19.5   META-ANALYSIS PLOTS

In more complex situations to understand heterogeneity and its sources, several graphs and diagrams have been established to use in meta-analysis.

19.5.1   FOREST PLOT

The forest plot is a graphical display of results of individual studies on a common scale. In this plot, the summary statistics are represented on the horizontal axis, and the individual studies are indicated on the vertical axis. The study results are represented by dots and their 95 percent confidence intervals by the lines joining them. A vertical line representing the weighted arithmetic mean of the end-points is also drawn. It allows a visual examination of the degree of heterogeneity between the study results.

Example: The forest plot showing prevalence rates of schizophrenia reported in 37 studies in India is as given figure 19.1.

19.5.2   FUNNEL PLOT

The funnel plot is a simple scatter plot of the end-points of individual/primary studies on the horizontal axis against the precision of the estimates on the vertical axis. The end-points from small studies will scatter more widely at the bottom of the graph, with the spread narrows among larger studies. In the absence of bias, this will resemble a symmetrical inverted funnel. Publication bias may lead to asymmetry in the funnel plot.

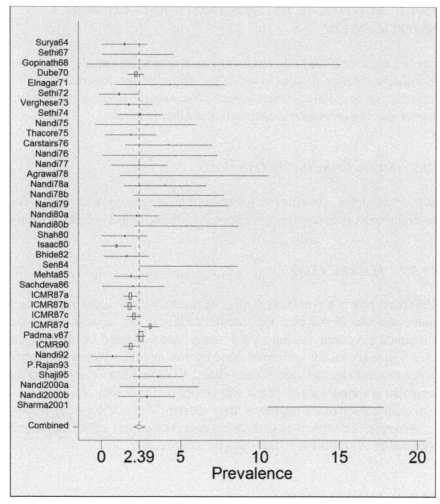

FIGURE 19.1   Forest plot showing prevalence rates of schizophrenia.

Example: The funnel plot for prevalence rates of schizophrenia reported in the 37 studies in India is as given given in figure 19.2.

FIGURE 19.2 Funnel plot showing prevalence rates of schizophrenia.

19.6 METHODS FOR POOLING END-POINTS: FIXED EFFECTS MODEL

The methods used to pool end-points employ a weighted average of the end-points in which the larger studies generally have more influence than the smaller ones. The methods are based on the assumption such as fixed effects model and random effects model.

19.6.1 FIXED EFFECTS MODEL

The fixed effects model assumes that there is only one population, and the variability between studies as due to random variation.

19.6.2 SAMPLE-SIZE METHOD

In this method, the weights for the studies are equal to their respective sample size (weighted arithmetic mean).

19.6.2.1   POOLED ESTIMATE

The pooled estimate is given by

$$\theta_{ss} = \frac{\sum n_i \theta_i}{\sum n_i}$$

where n_i is the sample size of the ith study.

19.6.3   INVERSE VARIANCE METHOD

The inverse variance (IV) method is used to pool either the binary, continuous, or correlation data. This approach has wide applicability since it can be used to combine any estimate that has standard error available. In this method, the weights for the studies are equal to their respective precisions of the estimates.

19.6.3.1   POOLED ESTIMATE

The pooled estimate is given by

$$\theta_{IV} = \frac{\sum w_i \theta_i}{\sum w_i}$$

where the weight w_i for the ith study is given by

$$w_i = \frac{1}{SE(\theta_i)^2}$$

The standard error of the pooled estimate is given by

$$SE(\theta_{IV}) = \frac{1}{\sqrt{w_i}}$$

19.6.4 HETEROGENEITY STATISTICS

The heterogeneity statistic of selected studies is given by

$$Q_w = \sum w_i (\theta_i - \theta_{IV})^2$$

where k is the number of studies included in the meta-analysis. The Q_w follows approximate chi-square distribution with df $= (k-1)$. Any significant heterogeneity between end-points found in the selected studies should not be considered as purely a problem for meta-analysis, since it provides an opportunity for examining why treatment effects differ in different circumstances. Careful investigation of the heterogeneity in meta-analysis should increase the scientific and clinical relevance.

19.7 METHODS FOR POOLING END-POINTS: RANDOM EFFECTS MODEL

19.7.1 RANDOM EFFECTS MODEL

The random effects model assumes that there are different populations and a different underlying effect for each study, and it takes this into account as an additional source of variation. The random effects models are used when there is considerable (significant) heterogeneity between end-points.

19.7.2 DL METHOD

The DL method (DerSimonian and Laird method) of meta-analysis is the commonly used random effects model method. The effect size θ_i is assumed to have a normal distribution with mean θ and variance τ^2.

19.7.2.1 POOLED ESTIMATE

In this method, the pooled estimate is given by

$$\theta_{DL} = \frac{\sum w_i^* \theta_i}{\sum w_i^*}$$

where the weight for the ith study is given by

$$w_i^* = \frac{1}{SE\left(\theta_i\right)^2 + \tau^2}$$

The variance of the studies is given by

$$\tau^2 = \frac{Q_w - (k-1)}{\sum w_i - \frac{\sum w_i^2}{\sum w_i}}$$

This is set to zero if $Q_w \leq (k-1)$. The standard error of the pooled estimate is given by

$$SE\left(\theta_{DL}\right) = \frac{1}{\sqrt{\sum w_i^*}}$$

19.8   ADDITIONAL META-ANALYSIS TECHNIQUES

It will be advantageous to extend meta-analysis by applying the following additional meta-analysis technique in order to draw important implications.

19.8.1   SENSITIVITY META-ANALYSIS TECHNIQUE

This technique is the study of influence of different statistical methodologies on the results of meta-analysis. The methodological issues include randomization versus non-randomization, random sampling versus non-random sampling, different sample size, fixed effects model versus random effects model, and different levels of quality assessments.

19.8.2   INFLUENCE META-ANALYSIS TECHNIQUE

In this technique, the influence of each study can be estimated by deleting each in turn from the analysis, and noticing down the degree of change in the pooled estimate and its level of significance.

19.8.3   SUB-GROUP META-ANALYSIS TECHNIQUE

The sub-group meta-analysis is the study of variation by different categories of patients on the results of meta-analysis. The estimate of the overall effect is intended to guide decisions about clinical practice for a wide range of patients. When the heterogeneity statistic is significant, it is not possible to assume that the given effect is same across different groups of treatments such as males versus females, young versus elderly, and those with mild versus those with severe diseases. It seems reasonable to base treatment decision upon the results of those studies that have similar characteristics to the particular patient under consideration.

19.8.4   CUMULATIVE META-ANALYSIS TECHNIQUE

This technique is a repeated performance of meta-analysis whenever a new relevant study is available for inclusion. This allows a retrospective identification of the patient in time whenever a treatment effect first reached conventional level of statistical significance. Subsequent studies will simply confirm the original results with reduced levels of significance. Further studies in large number of patients involving high cost may be avoided by conducting timely cumulative meta-analysis.

19.9   IMPLICATIONS OF THE RESULTS OF META-ANALYSIS

19.9.1   RESEARCH IMPLICATIONS

The meta-analysis helps scientists to plan new research.

19.9.2   CLINICAL IMPLICATIONS

The meta-analysis helps psychiatrists to produce evidence-based treatment. Applying results of meta-analysis to an individual patient involve consideration of the applicability of the evidence, the feasibility of the intervention in a particular settings, the risk ratio in the individual patient, and incorporation of patients' value and preferences.

19.9.3   ECONOMIC IMPLICATIONS

The meta-analysis helps in the development of methods for economic evaluation. The major implications of meta-analysis lies in the determination of the number needed to treat (NNT). The NNT is the number of patients that must be treated over a defined time period to prevent one death or disorder. Hence, it is the reciprocal of the risk difference (RD). That is,

$$NNT= \frac{1}{RD}$$

Thus, the NNT is commonly used to summarize the beneficial effect of treatment in a clinically relevant way.

19.9.4   IMPLICATIONS FOR POLICY MAKING

The meta-analysis helps policy makers to make meaningful decisions. Policy making should be based on best current knowledge and takes into account of resources and values in the interpretation of evidence.

19.9.5   NUMERICAL DEMONSTRATION

Let suppose that we have information on proportion of schizophrenia registrations at three mental institutes (hospitals) as shown in the following meta-analysis master sheet:

Mental institute	Ownership	Registrations	Schizophrenia	Proportion
A	private	91	8	0.0879
B	government	100	25	0.2500
C	private	109	5	0.0459
Combined	-	300	38	0.1270

We wish to obtain the pooled proportion of schizophrenia in these hospitals. As a first step, we have the weighted proportion based on sample-size method, as 0.127 or 12.7 percent. In order to apply the IV method of fixed effects model, we will have the computation table as shown below:

Institute	n	x	θ_i	$SE(\theta_i)^2$	w_i	θ_i	$(\theta_i-\theta_w)^2$
A	91	8	0.0879	.00088	1136	100	0.022
B	100	25	0.2500	.00188	532	133	14.748
C	109	5	0.0459	.00040	2500	115	3.534
Combined	300	38	0.1267	-	4168	348	18.304

$$\theta_{IV} = \frac{348}{4168} = 0.0835, \text{ that is, } 8.35\%$$

$$SE(\theta_{IV}) = \frac{1}{\sqrt{4168}} = \frac{1}{64.56} = 0.0155$$

From the table, the heterogeneity statistic is given as follows:

$Q_w = 18.304$ with df=2

Since the calculated value is more than the table value of $\chi^2(2) = 9.21$, the null hypothesis is rejected ($P<0.01$, highly significant). This means the hospitals are significantly different proportions of schizophrenic cases based on ownership. Hence, we may proceed with random effects model method such as the DL method. The variance of the end-points (proportion of schizophrenic cases) of the three hospitals is calculated to be as follows:

$$\tau^2 = \frac{18.304 - (3-1)}{4168 - (\frac{7823520}{4168})} = \frac{16.304}{2291} = 0.0071$$

The computation table for DL method is as given below:

Institute	n	x	θ_I	v_i	$v_i + \tau^2$	w_i^*	$\theta_I w_i^*$
(1)	(2)	(3)	(4)	(5)	(6)	(7)	(8)
A	91	8	0.0879	.00088	.00798	125	11.00
B	100	25	0.2500	.00188	.00898	111	27.75
C	109	5	0.0459	.00040	.00750	133	6.10
Combined	300	38	0.1267	-	-	369	44.85

$$\theta_{DL} = \frac{44.85}{369} = 0.1215 \text{ or } 12.15\%$$

$$SE(\theta_{DL}) = \frac{1}{\sqrt{369}} = 0.0521$$

Thus, the pooled estimate of proportion of schizophrenia registrations of mental hospitals are 0.1270 (based on sample size method), 0.0835 (based on IV method), 0.1215 (based on DL method). Since the heterogeneity statistic is significant, we have to accept the pooled estimate based on DL method.

KEYWORDS

- **End-points**
- **Heterogeneity statistics**
- **Meta-analysis**

CHAPTER 20

REPORTING THE RESULTS

CONTENTS

20.1   EVALUATION OF THE STUDY

20.1.1   DATA DESCRIPTION

- The study design must be appropriate to the objectives of the study. It depends on whether intervention is involved or not.
- The target population and the sampling units/observational units must be clearly defined, and suitable sampling method must be chosen.
- The sample size must be adequate to detect the difference/relationship that we look for. That is, we should provide adequate means of precision of the estimate.
- We must have all relevant explanatory variables. The outcome variable must be clearly defined.
- The rate of missing values/non-compliance must be reasonably low. The bias that is introduced must be determined.

20.1.2   INTERNAL VALIDITY AND EXTERNAL VALIDITY

Internal validity concerns observational bias, effect of random variation, outcome variation with the magnitude of the source, strength of relationship between source of exposure and outcome, and time relationship, whereas external validity concerns the applicability of the results to target population.

20.1.3   COMPARISON WITH OTHER EVIDENCES

The consistency of the results with those of other studies as well as the plausibility of the results must be specified.

20.2   INTERPRETING THE RESULTS

In confirmatory studies, strong conclusions can be drawn about the relationships found. Otherwise, it is only exploratory and further studies become necessary.

20.2.1   DATASET

- In experimental trials, one must consider the extent to which the subjects of some larger population are represented. However, this question does not arise in observational studies.
- Random sampling errors have decreasing importance as the sample size increases, bias does not.
- Important explanatory variables may produce outliers, which should not be missed. Confounding factors are operating that have not been unaccounted for.

20.2.2   DESCRIPTIVE STATISTICS

- The average values are not necessarily normal or typical values. The variability is also essential. In the same way, a regression line cannot be interpreted as meaning that most or all individuals would be expected to lie on it.
- The standard deviation is a direct estimate of variability in the population, whereas the standard error is a description of the precision of some estimate.

20.2.3   STATISTICAL INFERENCE

- Rejecting a null hypothesis does not mean that the alternate hypothesis is true.
- The statistical significance depends on sample size, not on scientific importance; with a large enough sample, you can detect the uninteresting minimal difference.
- In experimental studies, randomization of treatment assignments is supposed to guarantee that you can draw causal conclusions. In observational studies, we can only support causality on nonstatistical grounds. The important points that are to be considered include the strength of association between source of exposure and response, the consistency of association among different circumstances, people, place, and time; and the scientific plausibility of the explanations.
- In comparing your results with those previously obtained elsewhere, be careful about publication bias; only studies yielding statistically

significant results are generally published. One convenient method of comparing all studies on a subject is through an overview or meta-analysis.

20.3 WRITING THE REPORT

Your report will have the potentials to change what scientists or decision makers believe about the phenomenon under study. To make this possible, your report must
- be reasonably brief
- avoid long and technical words
- be well organized and coherent
- be in the form of tables and graphs where necessary
- ensure that reading your report should be a stimulating and satisfying experience

20.3.1 MAJOR CRITICISMS

The report should modify the scientific belief by strengthening, weakening or altering existing ones, or creating new ones. For this, the design or analysis should not be flawed. Major criticism will include the following:
- Unrepresentative sample to allow generalization
- Lack of or inadequate randomization
- Key missing explanatory variables.

20.3.2 WRITING SCIENTIFIC PAPERS

The publications in scientific journals will enable your results to be rapidly disseminated throughout the World. Never publish interim results of your experimental trials if the trial is continuing. This can bias the response still to come. In a properly designed study, the so-called negative findings of no relationship among key variables can be as important as positive ones. They do not indicate failure of the study. The basic sections of scientific papers are the following:
- Title
- Abstract (summary of your main results)

- Introduction (recalling relevant previous research and justifying your objectives in the present work)
- Method (describing what you do. That is, the protocol and how you followed it)
- Results (describe what you discovered)
- Discussion (interpreting your results and drawing implications)
- References (related publications in the field)
- Appendix (containing more technical and detailed supporting material)

20.3.3   WRITING TECHNICAL REPORTS

Many studies are conducted in order to make policy decision, whether in government or in private industry. The drive to produce valid and objective results may be much stronger than in scientific publishing because concrete action will be taken. The basic sections of technical papers are the following:
- Title
- Material and methods (study design and statistical model)
- Results (analysis and presentation)
- Discussion (interpretation)

All sections, except the discussion that gives the authors opinion, are supposed to be objective. Most readers will want to master the main results, and the nature of the arguments, along with its limitations.

20.3.4   REPORTING THE DATA ANALYSIS

- Give good reasons for excluding outlying observation.
- In case of estimation of parameters, generally avoid tests in favour of intervals of precision.
- Report all the tests made, not just the significance ones; otherwise, you are committing fraud.
- A statistically significant results neither mean that it is of any practical importance, nor does it even prove that the relationship is real.

20.3.5   *REPORTING THE RESULTS*

- Give the characteristics of non-respondents and dropouts. In experimental trials, thoroughly document and discuss both noncompliance and side effects from the intervention.
- In experimental trials, describe objectively what happened to subject on each treatment. In regression line, show all the individual observational points.
- The simple descriptive statistics may serve to illustrate results from more complex analysis that the general reader cannot be expected to understand. However, clearly document those complex analyses.
- The graphs and diagrams may be more useful along with the descriptive statistics. The important graphs and diagrams are given below:

> *Histogram* in one-variable descriptive statistics
> *Scatter plot* in correlation analysis
> *Regression line* in regression analysis
> *Survival curve* in survival analysis
> *Sequence chart* in time series analysis
> *Profiles* in multivariate analysis
> *Dendrogram* in cluster analysis
> *Screeplot* in factor analysis
> *Forest plot* in meta-analysis

KEYWORDS

- **Descriptive statistics**
- **Experimental trials**

CHAPTER 21

STATISTICAL PACKAGE FOR SOCIAL SCIENCES

CONTENTS

21.1   SPSS DATA EDITOR

Once installed, SPSS can be opened like any other windows-based application by clicking on the start menu at the bottom left-hand corner of the screen and by clicking on SPSS for windows from the list of programs; or by clicking on the icon on the screen. This activates the SPSS data editor window as shown in the following figure.

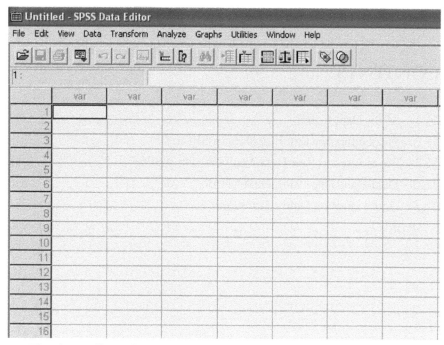

The data editor (data view) window is the main data editor where all the data are entered much like an Excel spreadsheet.

21.1.1   MENU ITEMS

At the top of the screen, there are different menus that give access to various functions of SPSS. This consists of 10 menus, which provides access to every tool of the SPSS program.

21.1.1.1   FILE, EDIT, AND VIEW

The file menu lets us open, save, print, and close file and provides access to recently used files, etc. The Edit menu allows us do things such as copy, cut, paste, etc. The View menu can hide or show the toolbar, status bar, gridlines, etc.

21.1.1.2   DATA AND TRANSFORM

The Data menu allows us to manipulate the data in various ways. We can define variables, go to a particular case, sort cases, transpose them, merge cases, as well as variables from some other file. We can also select cases on which we want to run the analysis and split the file to arrange the output of analysis in a particular manner. The Transform menu lets us compute new variables and make changes to existing ones.

21.1.1.3   ANALYZE AND GRAPH

The Analyze menu is the function that lets us perform all the statistical analysis. This has various statistical tools grouped under different categories. The Graph menu lets us make various types of plots from our data.

21.1.1.4   UTILITIES, WINDOW, AND HELP

The Utilities menu gives us information about variables and files. Finally, the Window and Help menus are very similar to other windows application menus.

21.1.2   FURTHER ITEMS

Below the menu bar, there is a toolbar that has buttons for quick access to various functions. The same functions can be performed by choosing relevant options from the menus. There are 17 items in the tool bar - Open, Save, Print, Recall Dialogue, etc. At the bottom of the screen, we have a status bar like SPSS is ready. The program can be closed by clicking on the close button at the top right-hand side corner.

21.2 PROCEDURES FOR ENTERING DATA IN SPSS

As shown in SPSS data editor window, the bottom of the data editor has two tabs: data view and variable view. When in data view, the data editor works pretty much in the same manner as an Excel spread sheet. One can enter values in different cells, modifying them, and even cut and paste to and from an Excel spread sheet. When the data editor is in variable view, the data editor window is as shown below:

	Name	Type	Width	Decimals	Label	Values	Missing	Columns	Align	Measure
1	regn	Numeric	8	0		None	None	8	Right	Scale
2	serial	Numeric	8	0		None	None	8	Right	Scale
3	age	Numeric	8	0		None	None	8	Right	Scale
4	sex	Numeric	8	0		{1, male}...	None	8	Right	Scale
5	maritals	Numeric	8	0		{1, single}...	None	8	Right	Scale
6	locality	Numeric	8	0		{1, rural}...	None	8	Right	Scale
7	icd10	Numeric	8	1		None	None	8	Right	Scale
8										
9										
10										

osdata - SPSS Data Editor

File Edit View Data Transform Analyze Graphs Utilities Window Help

In addition to entering the values of the variables, we have to provide information about them in SPSS. This can be done when the data editor is in variable view. Notice that there are 10 columns in the data editor (variable view) window. We will explain the use of each of these 10 columns in entering the data with the help of the data of 40 psychiatric patients as shown in Appendix I.

21.2.1 NAME

In our example, we have seven variables to enter. We will name registration number as "regn," serial number of the patients as "serial," age and sex can be named as it is, marital status as "marital," and so on.

21.2.2   TYPE, WIDTH, AND DECIMAL

The second column titled "type" lets us define the variable type. If we click on the cell next to variable name and in the type column, a dialogue box appears as shown in figure below.

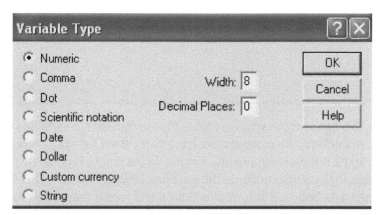

The most common type used is numeric, which means that the variable has a numeric value. The other common choice is string, which means that the available is in test format. We cannot perform any statistical analysis on a numeric variable if it is specified as a string variable. Since our variables are of numeric type, we select numeric from the dialogue box as shown in the figure above. We can also specify the width of the variable column and decimal places on this dialogue box.

21.2.3   VALUE AND LABEL

We have a column titled "label." Here, we can write the details about a particular variable in this column. We have a column labeled "values." If we click on the cell next to the variable name and in the values columns, a dialogue box appears as shown in the figure below.

In this box, we can specify values for our qualitative variables (categories). In our data, for example, we have two values for sex: 1 representing male and 2 representing female. Enter 1 in the empty box labeled "value" and specify its name (male) in the next box labeled "value." This will activate the Add button. Click on this button and repeat these steps to specify female.

21.2.4   FURTHER ITEMS

We have a column labeled "missing" to specify missing values. By default, no missing value is selected here. The next column titled "column" helps us modify the way we wish to view the data on screen. In this column, the width of the column can be specified. In the Align column, we can specify if we want our data to be right, left, or center aligned. Finally, in the column titled "measure," we can specify whether our variable is nominal, ordinal, or scale (interval or ratio).

21.2.5   SAVING THE FILE

Once the variables are specified, we can switch to data view and enter the data. This data file can be saved just as MS Word file and reopened by double clicking on the file from its saved location. The data in Appendix I are as shown below in the data editor:

data - SPSS Data Editor

File Edit View Data Transform Analyze Graphs Utilities Window Help

1 : regn   293307

	regn	serial	age	sex	maritals	locality	icd10	var
1	293307	1	60	1	2	1	32.3	
2	293308	2	80	2	1	1	.1	
3	293309	3	4	2	1	3	80.0	
4	293310	4	22	2	1	1	34.0	
5	293311	5	26	1	2	1	23.0	
6	293312	6	21	1	1	1	20.3	
7	293313	7	23	2	2	1	32.3	
8	293314	8	25	1	1	1	20.3	
9	293315	9	29	1	2	3	42.0	
10	293316	10	9	2	1	3	81.3	
11	293317	11	51	1	2	1	44.5	
12	293318	12	31	2	2	2	34.1	
13	293319	13	48	2	2	1	41.1	
14	293320	14	25	2	1	1	32.3	
15	293321	15	65	1	2	2	29.0	
16	293322	16	12	1	1	1	81.3	
17	293323	17	16	2	1	1	70.0	
18	293324	18	13	1	1	3	70.0	
19	293325	19	29	1	2	3	31.1	
20	293326	20	76	1	2	1	31.4	
21	293327	21	12	1	1	2	90.0	
22	293328	22	10	1	1	1	81.3	
23	293329	23	35	1	2	2	10.3	
24	293330	24	40	1	2	2	20.0	
25	293331	25	11	1	1	3	44.9	
26	293332	26	70	1	2	3	31.0	
27	293333	27	24	2	1	3	43.0	
28	293334	28	58	2	2	2	.0	
29	293335	29	60	2	2	2	23.0	
30	293336	30	27	1	1	2	30.1	
31	293337	31	30	1	1	2	43.2	
32	293338	32	50	2	1	1	29.0	
33	293339	33	26	1	1	2	31.0	
34	293340	34	25	1	1	2	29.0	
35	293341	35	27	1	1	3	42.0	
36	293342	36	19	1	1	3	31.8	
37	293343	37	33	2	2	3	33.0	
38	293344	38	35	1	1	1	34.1	
39	293345	39	24	2	2	2	31.6	
40	293346	40	44	2	2	2	33.1	

21.3   PROCEDURES TO RUN DATA ANALYSIS USING SPSS

21.3.1   DATASET AND DATA EDITOR FORMAT

The dataset to be analyzed will be with the researcher in his own format. Usually, the format will be that the subjects (patients) are represented by the rows and the variables will be represented by the columns. The data editor formats are different for different statistical method. Let us suppose that we have the data as shown in Appendix I.

21.3.2   PLAN OF ANALYSIS

The researcher has to note down as to how many cases, how many variables, and the level of measurement of each variable. The researcher must have a plan of analysis (statistical methods to be applied) and an idea of the appropriate dialogue box in the particular version of SPSS. In order to select appropriate dialogue box, click on Analyze, which will produce a dropdown menu. The Analyze menu includes descriptive statistics, compare means, etc. Let us wish to obtain frequency distribution of diagnosis (ICD-10) variable for our data. The data are entered in the data editor with an appropriate data editor format as shown above.

21.3.3   MAIN DIALOGUE BOX

Since we have planned to obtain frequencies of diagnosis variable, select *descriptive statistics* and then click on *Frequencies*, which will produce the dialogue box as shown in the figure below.

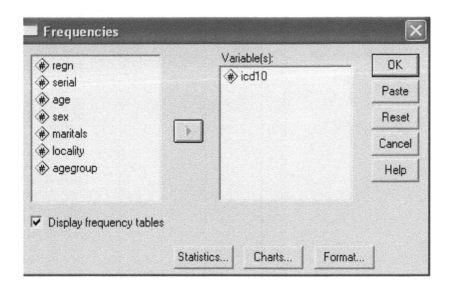

21.3.4   OUTPUT

In this dialogue box, we have to select the variables for which we wish to obtain frequencies, by transferring them to the variables box on the right-hand side from the left-hand side box. For this, first highlight the variable: ICD-10 by clicking on it. Then, click on the arrow button between the two boxes. The highlighted variable will get transferred to the other box. There are some default selections made in this box about the statistics to be shown in the output. A particular statistic can be selected or deselected for display in the output by clicking on the box next to their names. We have not selected any additional statistics other than what is selected by default. Click on OK to run the analysis.

Whenever we run any command in SPSS, the output is shown in the SPSS viewer, which opens as a separate window. The SPSS viewer window has two panels. The right-hand side panel shows the active output and the left-hand side panel shows an outline of the output shown in the right-hand side panel. One can quickly navigate through the output by selecting the same from the outline provided in the left-hand side panel. The requisite output for our data is as given below:

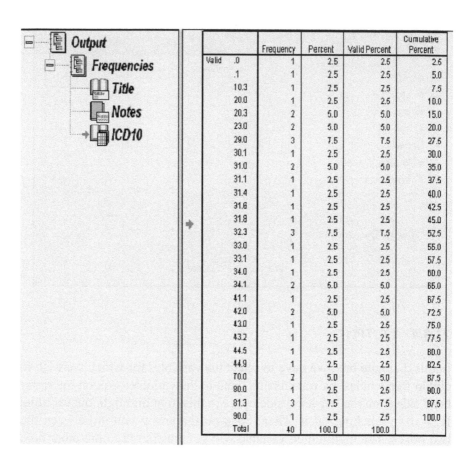

		Frequency	Percent	Valid Percent	Cumulative Percent
Valid	.0	1	2.5	2.5	2.5
	.1	1	2.5	2.5	5.0
	10.3	1	2.5	2.5	7.5
	20.0	1	2.5	2.5	10.0
	20.3	2	5.0	5.0	15.0
	23.0	2	5.0	5.0	20.0
	29.0	3	7.5	7.5	27.5
	30.1	1	2.5	2.5	30.0
	31.0	2	5.0	5.0	35.0
	31.1	1	2.5	2.5	37.5
	31.4	1	2.5	2.5	40.0
	31.6	1	2.5	2.5	42.5
	31.8	1	2.5	2.5	45.0
	32.3	3	7.5	7.5	52.5
	33.0	1	2.5	2.5	55.0
	33.1	1	2.5	2.5	57.5
	34.0	1	2.5	2.5	60.0
	34.1	2	5.0	5.0	65.0
	41.1	1	2.5	2.5	67.5
	42.0	2	5.0	5.0	72.5
	43.0	1	2.5	2.5	75.0
	43.2	1	2.5	2.5	77.5
	44.5	1	2.5	2.5	80.0
	44.9	1	2.5	2.5	82.5
	70.0	2	5.0	5.0	87.5
	80.0	1	2.5	2.5	90.0
	81.3	3	7.5	7.5	97.5
	90.0	1	2.5	2.5	100.0
	Total	40	100.0	100.0	

Output
Frequencies
Title
Notes
ICD10

21.4   DATA HANDLING USING DATA MENU

The commands described in the data menu are very useful for managing large and complex data files. The commands in data menu include select cases, weight cases, etc.

21.4.1   SPLIT FILE

Researchers may need to run analysis on a subject of the cases from the existing variables based on certain conditions. The split file commands temporarily split the file into groups. All the analysis done after splitting a file will be done separately on different subgroups, and the output will be arranged according to these groups. For example, in our data in the data editor format, we wish to obtain the frequencies of males and females separately; we have to split the file by this variable. Click on Data Menu in the data editor window and select *Split File* from the dropdown menu.

21.4.1.1   MAIN DIALOGUE BOX

The split file commands are as shown in the figure below:

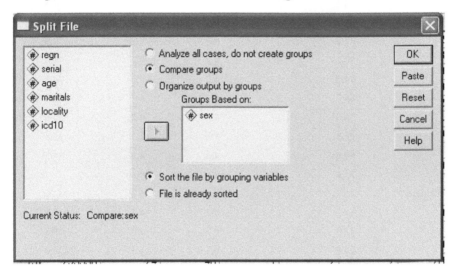

The default option in the window is to analyze all cases, do not create groups. The other options are select compare groups or organize output by groups. Selecting either of these will activate the box labeled groups based on. Select sex and transfer to this box. Click on OK to complete splitting the file. Now, if you run any analysis, two outputs will be produced, one for each of the categories. We wish to obtain the frequency distribution of diagnosis (ICD-10) according to sex. The result is as given below:

SEX	ICD-10	Frequency	Percent	Valid percent	Cumulative percent
Male	10.3	1	4.2	4.2	4.2
	20.0	1	4.2	4.2	8.3
	20.3	2	8.3	8.3	16.7
	23.0	1	4.2	4.2	20.8

SEX	ICD-10	Frequency	Percent	Valid percent	Cumulative percent
	29.0	2	8.3	8.3	29.2
	30.1	1	4.2	4.2	33.3
	31.0	2	8.3	8.3	41.7
	31.1	1	4.2	4.2	45.8
	31.4	1	4.2	4.2	50.0
	31.8	1	4.2	4.2	54.2
	32.3	1	4.2	4.2	58.3
	34.1	1	4.2	4.2	62.5
	42.0	2	8.3	8.3	70.8
	43.2	1	4.2	4.2	75.0
	44.5	1	4.2	4.2	79.2
	44.9	1	4.2	4.2	83.3
	70.0	1	4.2	4.2	87.5
	81.3	2	8.3	8.3	95.8
	90.0	1	4.2	4.2	100.0
	Total	24	100.0	100.0	
Female	.0	1	6.3	6.3	6.3
	.1	1	6.3	6.3	12.5
	23.0	1	6.3	6.3	18.8
	29.0	1	6.3	6.3	25.0
	31.6	1	6.3	6.3	31.3
	32.3	2	12.5	12.5	43.8
	33.0	1	6.3	6.3	50.0
	33.1	1	6.3	6.3	56.3
	34.0	1	6.3	6.3	62.5
	34.1	1	6.3	6.3	68.8
	41.1	1	6.3	6.3	75.0
	43.0	1	6.3	6.3	81.3
	70.0	1	6.3	6.3	87.5
	80.0	1	6.3	6.3	93.8
	81.3	1	6.3	6.3	100.0
	Total	16	100.0	100.0	-

Spitting file is a temporary option and you can cancel it by selecting analyze all cases, do not create groups.

21.4.2 WEIGHT CASES

Sometimes, the researcher may want to carry out, for example, chi-square test of significance from the frequencies in the contingency table. In such cases, the "weight cases" command in the data menu has to be used. Let us demonstrate this by a 2 × 2 contingency table as shown below:

Sex	Single	Married	Total
Male	14	10	24
Female	7	9	16
Total	21	19	40

The frequencies in 2 × 2 contingency table are entered as shown in the following data editor, where the rows (sex) and columns (marital status) are specified.

21.4.2.1   MAIN DIALOGUE BOX

Now, click on OK, which will produce a dropdown menu, choose weight cases from that, and click on the OK button.

Now, click on Analyze, choose *descriptive statistics* and click on crosstab. The rows and columns are entered in their respective boxes, and now click on the OK button to run the analysis. The requisite output extracted is as shown below:

Chi-Square Tests

	Value	df	Asymp. Sig. (2-sided)	Exact Sig. (2-sided)	Exact Sig. (1-sided)
Pearson Chi-Square	.819[b]	1	.366		
Continuity Correction[a]	.338	1	.561		
Likelihood Ratio	.820	1	.365		
Fisher's Exact Test				.520	.281
Linear-by-Linear Association	.798	1	.372		
N of Valid Cases	40				

a. Computed only for a 2x2 table

b. 0 cells (.0%) have expected count less than 5. The minimum expected count is 7.60.

21.5   DATA HANDLING USING TRANSFORM MENU

21.5.1   RECODE

Sometimes, we may want to recode some of the variables. For example, we may want to create categories of age with 10 years' interval. Click on *Transform* in the data editor window and select Recode from the drop-down menu as shown in the figure below.

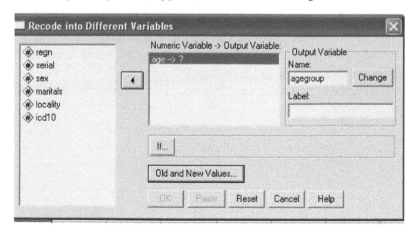

Click on *"Into Different Variables"* that produces a dialogue box. Select age and transfer it into the box labeled input–output variable. Once this is done, two boxes on the left-hand side become active. We have to specify the name and label of the new variable in these boxes. Type age in that box labeled "name" and "age group" as its label in the box labeled "label." Now click on the button labeled "change" to transfer the name of the output variable into the box labeled "input variable–output variable."

21.5.1.1   MAIN DIALOGUE BOX

The resulting dialogue box appears as shown in the figure below:

Next, click on the boxes labeled "Old and New Values," which produces a dialogue box as shown in the figure below. In this box, we have
to specify our recoding strategy, which is to recode age. Specify the first
range, zero through 9, specify zero in the box "New Value." Click on Add
to transfer these values to the box labeled Old-->New. In a similar manner,
specify the second range in the box range 10 through 19, specify 1 in the
box New Value. Click on Add to transfer these values to the box labeled
Old-->New, and so on. The resulting dialogue box is as shown in the figure below.

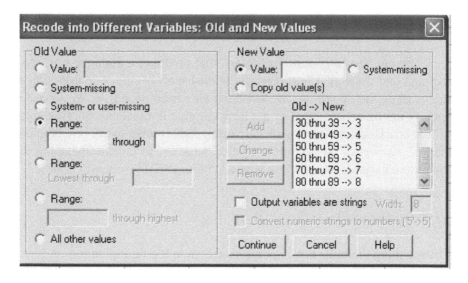

Click on "Continue" to return to the main dialogue box. Click on the
OK button to complete the recoding exercise. A new variable named "age
group" is created in the data file, which takes values 0, 1, 2, 3, etc. for age
groups. After running on the new data editor for frequencies, the output is
as shown below:

AGEGROUP

		Frequency	Percent	Valid Percent	Cumulative Percent
Valid	.00	2	5.0	5.0	5.0
	1.00	7	17.5	17.5	22.5
	2.00	14	35.0	35.0	57.5
	3.00	5	12.5	12.5	70.0
	4.00	3	7.5	7.5	77.5
	5.00	3	7.5	7.5	85.0
	6.00	3	7.5	7.5	92.5
	7.00	2	5.0	5.0	97.5
	8.00	1	2.5	2.5	100.0
	Total	40	100.0	100.0	

KEYWORDS

- **Data editor**
- **Data-handing**
- **Descriptive statistics**
- **ICD-10**
- **SPSS**

RUNNING DATA ANALYSIS USING SPSS

CONTENTS

22.1   RUNNING "PARAMETRIC TESTS OF SIGNIFICANCE" (METHODS IN CHAPTER 9)

22.1.1   RUNNING "ONE-SAMPLE *t*-TEST"

Let us suppose that the improvement scores of a group of five patients are as given in the following data editor:

▦ Untitled - SPSS Data Editor						
File Edit View Data Transform Analyze Graphs Utilities Window Help						
13:						
	patient	score	var	var	var	var
1	1	7				
2	2	4				
3	3	1				
4	4	3				
5	5	5				
6						
7						

We wish to test whether the mean score of all the patients can be assumed as 5.0.

22.1.1.1   MAIN DIALOGUE BOX

Click on *analyze* menu, which will produce dropdown menu. Choose *compare means* from that and click on *one-sample t-test*. The resultant dialogue box is as shown below. In the dialogue box, the variable (score) is selected for analysis by transferring them to the test variable box on the right-hand side. Next, change the value in the test value box, which originally appears as zero to the one against which we are testing the sample mean. In this case, the value would be 5.0.

Click on the OK button to run the analysis. The output produced is as shown in the following table.

One-Sample Statistics

	N	Mean	Std. Deviation	Std. Error Mean
SCORE	5	4.00	2.236	1.000

One-Sample Test

	Test Value = 5					
					95% Confidence Interval of the Difference	
	t	df	Sig. (2-tailed)	Mean Difference	Lower	Upper
SCORE	-1.000	4	.374	-1.00	-3.78	1.78

22.1.2   RUNNING "INDEPENDENT SAMPLES t-TEST"

Let us suppose that the improvement scores of experimental patients group and a control group patient are as given in the following data editor. In the data editor, we have codes for the two groups: 1 representing the control group and 2 representing the experimental group.

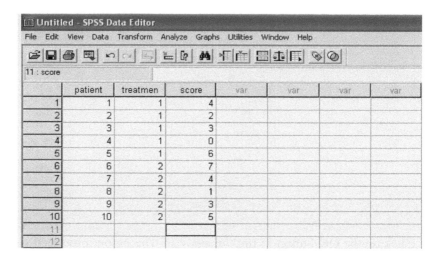

We wish to test whether the mean scores of the two groups are significantly different.

22.1.2.1   MAIN DIALOGUE BOX

Click on *analyze*, which will produce a dropdown menu, choose *compare means* from that, and click on *independent sample t-test*. The resultant dialogue box is as shown below:

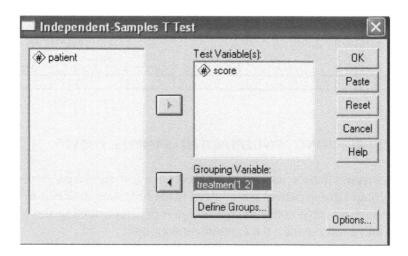

To perform independent sample *t*-test, transform dependent variable (score) into the test variable box and transfer the variable that identifies the groups (dependent) into the grouping variable box. Once the grouping variable is transferred, the "define groups" button which was earlier inactive turns active. Clicking on it will produce a box as shown below:

In our example, group 1 represents the control group and group 2 represents the experimental group, which we have entered under the variable group in the data editor. Therefore, put 1 in the box against group 1 and put 2 in the box against group 2, and click on "Continue." Now, click on the OK button to run the analysis. The output produced is as shown in the following table.

Independent Samples Test

		Levene's Test for Equality of Variances		t-test for Equality of Means						
									95% Confidence Interval of the Difference	
		F	Sig.	t	df	Sig. (2-tailed)	Mean Difference	Std. Error Difference	Lower	Upper
SCORE	Equal variances assumed	.000	1.000	-.707	8	.500	-1.00	1.414	-4.261	2.261
	Equal variances not assumed			-.707	8.000	.500	-1.00	1.414	-4.261	2.261

22.1.3 RUNNING "PAIRED-SAMPLE t-TEST"

The scores obtained by a group of five patients before giving the treatment, and the scores obtained by the patients after giving the treatment are given in the following data editor.

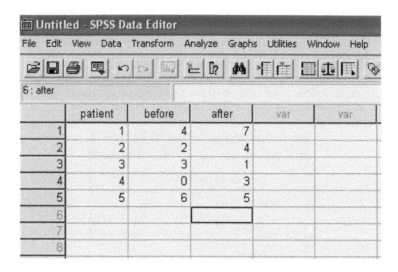

We wish to test whether the treatment program has significantly improved.

22.1.3.1   MAIN DIALOGUE BOX

Click on *analyze,* which will produce a dropdown menu, choose *compare means* from that, and click on *paired-sample t-test.* The resultant dialogue box is as shown below:

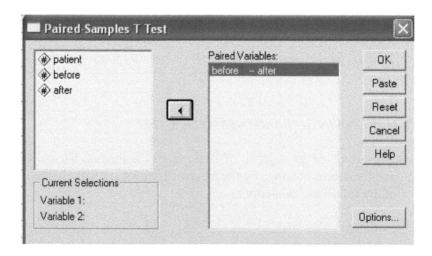

The variables to be compared (before, after) are transferred to the right-hand side box named paired variables. They will appear as before–after. Click on the OK button to run the analysis. The output produced is shown in the following fable.

Paired Samples Test

		Paired Differences							
					95% Confidence Interval of the Difference				
		Mean	Std. Deviation	Std. Error Mean	Lower	Upper	t	df	Sig. (2-tailed)
Pair 1	BEFORE - AFTER	-1.00	2.345	1.049	-3.91	1.91	-.953	4	.394

22.2 RUNNING "ANOVA TESTS" (METHODS IN CHAPTER 10)

22.2.1 RUNNING "ONE-WAY ANOVA"

The scores obtained by 15 patients from three treatment programs using a CRD are as given in the following data editor. We have three values for treatment:1 representing treatment 1,2 representing treatment 2, and 3 representing treatment 3.

	patient	treat	score
1	1	1	4
2	2	1	2
3	3	1	3
4	4	1	0
5	5	1	6
6	6	2	7
7	7	2	4
8	8	2	1
9	9	2	3
10	10	2	5
11	11	3	10
12	12	3	7
13	13	3	8
14	14	3	6
15	15	3	4

We wish to test whether the mean scores of the three treatments are significantly different.

22.2.1.1   MAIN DIALOGUE BOX

Click on *analyze*, which will produce a dropdown menu, choose *compare means* from that, and click on *one-way ANOVA*. The resultant dialogue box is as shown in the following figure:

Transfer the variable score into the box labeled dependent list and the factoring variable (treatment) into the box labeled "Factor."

Click on OK to run the analysis. The output for one-way ANOVA is as shown below:

ANOVA

SCORE

	Sum of Squares	df	Mean Square	F	Sig.
Between Groups	43.333	2	21.667	4.333	.038
Within Groups	60.000	12	5.000		
Total	103.333	14			

22.2.2 RUNNING "ANCOVA TEST"

Let us suppose that the marks scored in a test by three groups of multipurpose workers before conducting a training program and the marks scored
by the group after conducting the training program are as shown in the
following table.

Group 1		Group 2		Group 3	
Before	After	Before	After	Before	After
4	4	6	7	8	10
2	2	5	4	6	7
1	3	3	1	9	8
0	0	3	3	8	6
3	6	8	5	4	4

The given data are entered in the data editor as shown below. The
variables are labeled student, group, before, and after. For grouping
variable:1 represents group1,2 represents group 2, and 3 represents group
3.

ancova data - SPSS Data Editor

File   Edit   View   Data   Transform   Analyze   Graphs   Utilities   Window   Help

16 : after

	group	before	after	var	var	var
1	1	4	4			
2	1	2	2			
3	1	1	3			
4	1	0	0			
5	1	3	6			
6	2	6	7			
7	2	5	4			
8	2	3	1			
9	2	3	3			
10	2	8	5			
11	3	8	10			
12	3	6	7			
13	3	9	8			
14	3	8	6			
15	3	4	4			

We wish to test the significance of mean scores after conducting the training program and after subtracting from each individual score that portion which is predictable from the concomitant variable.

22.2.2.1   MAIN DIALOGUE BOX

Click on a*nalyze*, which will produce a dropdown menu, choose *general linear model* from that and click *univariate*. The resultant dialogue box is as shown below.

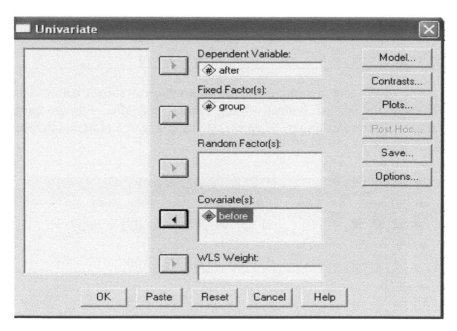

As shown in the above dialogue box, the group is transferred to the fixed factor box, the before is transferred to covariate box, and after is transferred to the dependent variable box. Now, click on the OK button to run the analysis.

The output is displayed in a table named "Tests of Between-Subjects Effects." We are interested only in the following results that are extracted from the table shown below.

Tests of Between-Subjects Effects

Dependent Variable: AFTER

Source	Type III Sum of Squares	df	Mean Square	F	Sig.
Corrected Model	76.152ᵃ	3	25.384	10.272	.002
Intercept	.721	1	.721	.292	.600
BEFORE	32.818	1	32.818	13.281	.004
GROUP	6.709	2	3.355	1.358	.297
Error	27.182	11	2.471		
Total	430.000	15			
Corrected Total	103.333	14			

a. R Squared = .737 (Adjusted R Squared = .665)

22.2.3 RUNNING "REPEATED MEASURES ANOVA"

The repeated measures scores of five students in three tests are as given in the following data editor:

	student	repeat1	repeat2	repeat3	var
1	1	4	7	10	
2	2	2	4	7	
3	3	3	1	8	
4	4	0	3	6	
5	5	6	5	4	
6					
7					

repeat ANOVA - SPSS Data Editor

File   Edit   View   Data   Transform   Analyze   Graphs   Utilities   Window   Help

6 : repeat3

We wish to test whether there is a significant improvement in these repetitions of the test by applying repeated ANOVA.

22.2.3.1 MAIN DIALOGUE BOX

Click on *analyze*, which will produce a dropdown menu, choose *general linear model* from that, and click on *repeated measures*. The resulting dialogue box is as shown below:

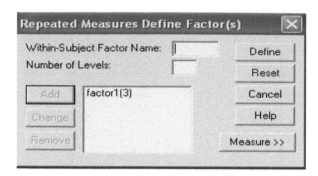

The number of levels (three in our example) is entered in the box "number of levels" as shown in the above-cited dialogue box. Then, "add" will be highlighted. Clicking on "add" will show factor(3)in the appropriate box. Click on "define" to produce the dialogue box as shown below:

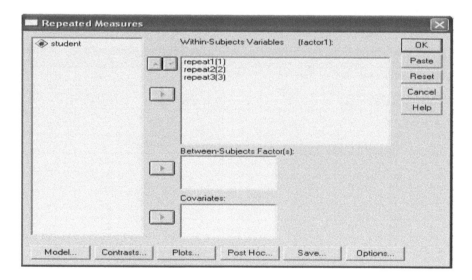

The three levels are transferred serially to the right-hand side box named Within-Subjects Variables (factor1). Click on OK to run the analysis. The SPSS display repeated ANOVA in many tables. We are interested in the following results:

Tests of Within-Subjects Effects

Measure: MEASURE_1

Source		Type III Sum of Squares	df	Mean Square	F	Sig.
FACTOR1	Sphericity Assumed	43.333	2	21.667	5.200	.036
	Greenhouse-Geisser	43.333	1.703	25.445	5.200	.046
	Huynh-Feldt	43.333	2.000	21.667	5.200	.036
	Lower-bound	43.333	1.000	43.333	5.200	.085
Error(FACTOR1)	Sphericity Assumed	33.333	8	4.167		
	Greenhouse-Geisser	33.333	6.812	4.893		
	Huynh-Feldt	33.333	8.000	4.167		
	Lower-bound	33.333	4.000	8.333		

22.3 RUNNING "NON-PARAMETRIC TESTS OF SIGNIFICANCE"(METHODS IN CHAPTER 11)

22.3.1 RUNNING "CHI-SQUARE TESTS OF SIGNIFICANCE"

The data regarding sex and marital status of the 40 registered psychiatric patients (data in Appendix I with one patient data on married is changed to single) is as presented in data editor format in Chapter 21.2.5. The variable sex has two categories: 1representing male and 2 representing female. Similarly, the variable marital status has two categories: 1 representing unmarried and 2 representing married.

We wish to test whether sex and marital status is independent or not, by running chi-square test of significance.

22.3.1.1 MAIN DIALOGUE BOX

Click on *analyze*, which will produce a dropdown menu, choose *descriptive statistics* from that, and click on *crosstab*. The resulting dialogue box appears as shown below:

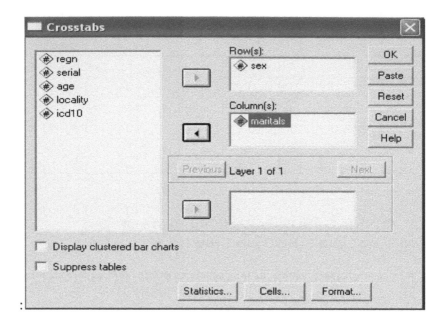

The sex is transferred to the box labeled column and marital status is transferred to the box labeled rows. Next, click on the statistics button that brings up a dialogue box. Select the first box labeled chi-square in this subdialogue box and click on "continue" button to return to the previous screen. Click on continue to return to the main dialogue box. Now, click on OK to run the analysis. The output produced will be as shown below:

SEX * MARITALS Crosstabulation

Count

		MARITALS		Total
		single	married	
SEX	male	14	10	24
	female	8	8	16
Total		22	18	40

Chi-Square Tests

	Value	df	Asymp. Sig. (2-sided)	Exact Sig. (2-sided)	Exact Sig. (1-sided)
Pearson Chi-Square	.269b	1	.604		
Continuity Correction a	.038	1	.846		
Likelihood Ratio	.269	1	.604		
Fisher's Exact Test				.748	.422
Linear-by-Linear Association	.263	1	.608		
N of Valid Cases	40				

a. Computed only for a 2x2 table

b. 0 cells (.0%) have expected count less than 5. The minimum expected count is 7.20.

22.3.2   RUNNING "RUN TEST"

The data regarding sex and marital status of the 40 registered psychiatric patients (data in Appendix I) are as presented in data editor format in Chapter 21.2.5. The variable sex has two categories: 1representing male and 2 representing female.

We wish to test whether there is a significant randomness in the occurrence of males and females in the sequence.

22.3.2.1   MAIN DIALOGUE BOX

Click on a*nalyze*, which will produce a dropdown menu, choose *non-parametric test* from that, and click on *runs*. The resultant dialogue box is as given below:

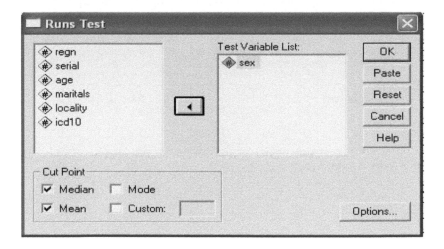

The variable sex is transferred to the box named "test variable list." The default selection for cut point is median. We have to select mean as the cut point in order to clearly distinguish between males and females. Now, click on OK to run the analysis. The requisite output is as given below:

Runs Test 2

	SEX
Test Value[a]	1.40
Cases < Test Value	24
Cases >= Test Value	16
Total Cases	40
Number of Runs	18
Z	-.568
Asymp. Sig. (2-tailed)	.570

a. Mean

22.3.3   RUNNING "MANN–WHITNEY U-TEST"

The marks scored in a test by 10 students from two departments are as given in the following data editor (1 representing the first department and 2 representing the second department).

mannd - SPSS Data Editor				
File Edit View Data Transform Analyze Graphs Utilities W					

1 : student		1		
	student	dept	score	var
1	1	1	4	
2	2	1	2	
3	3	1	3	
4	4	1	0	
5	5	1	6	
6	6	2	9	
7	7	2	7	
8	8	2	8	
9	9	2	5	
10	10	2	11	
11				
12				

We wish to test whether the median score of the students in the two departments are significantly different by using Mann–Whitney U-test.

22.3.3.1 MAIN DIALOGUE BOX

Click on *analyze*, which will produce a dropdown menu, choose *non-parametric tests* from that, and click *two-independent sample tests*. The resultant dialogue box is as given below:

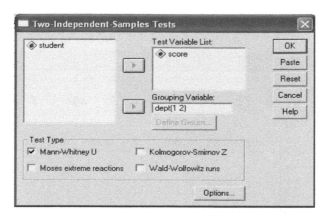

The variable score is transferred to the test variable list box. The department is transferred to the grouping variable box and defining groups by 1 and 2. Now, click on OK to run the analysis. The output is as given below:

Ranks

	DEPT	N	Mean Rank	Sum of Ranks
SCORE	1	5	3.20	16.00
	2	5	7.80	39.00
	Total	10		

Test Statistics[b]

	SCORE
Mann-Whitney U	1.000
Wilcoxon W	16.000
Z	-2.402
Asymp. Sig. (2-tailed)	.016
Exact Sig. [2*(1-tailed Sig.)]	.016[a]

a. Not corrected for ties.

b. Grouping Variable: DEPT

22.3.4   RUNNING "KRUSHKAL–WALLIS *H*-TEST"

The marks scored by 15 students in a test, from three departments are as given in the following data editor. The variables are labeled as shown in the following figure. We have three values for departments: 1 representing the first department, 2 representing the second department, and 3 representing the third department.

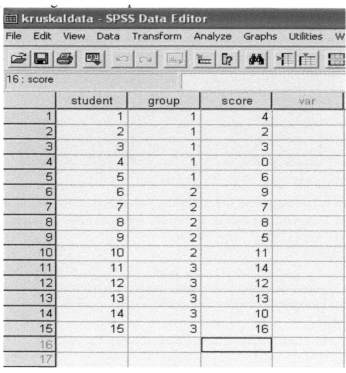

We wish to test whether the median scores of the student in three departments are same, by running the Krushkal–Wallis *H*-test.

22.3.4.1   *MAIN DIALOGUE BOX*

Click on *analyze* menu, which will produce a dropdown menu, choose *non-parametric tests* from that, and click on *tests for several independent-samples*. The resultant dialogue box is as shown below:

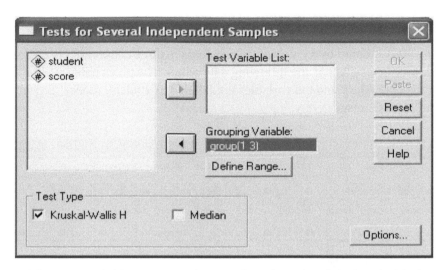

The test variables (scores) is transferred to the right-hand side box named "test variable list." The department is transferred to the grouping variable box. Define the range as 1–3 in the subdialogue box. Now, click on OK to run the analysis. The output is as given below:

Kruskal-Wallis Test

Ranks

	GROUP	N	Mean Rank
SCORE	1	5	3.20
	2	5	8.00
	3	5	12.80
	Total	15	

Test Statistics[a,b]

	SCORE
Chi-Square	11.520
df	2
Asymp. Sig.	.003

a. Kruskal Wallis Test

b. Grouping Variable: GROUP

22.3.5   RUNNING "FRIEDMAN TEST"

The marks scored by a group of five students in three consecutively repeated tests are as given in the following data editor. The given data are entered in the data editor and the variables are labeled as student, repeat1, repeat2, and repeat3, respectively.

	student	repeat1	repeat2	repeat3	var	var
1	1	4	7	10		
2	2	2	4	7		
3	3	3	1	8		
4	4	0	3	6		
5	5	6	5	4		
6						
7						

friedmandata - SPSS Data Editor

File   Edit   View   Data   Transform   Analyze   Graphs   Utilities   Window   Help

1 : student   1

We wish to test whether there is a significant improvement in these repetitions of the test.

22.3.5.1   MAIN DIALOGUE BOX

Click on *analyze*, which will produce a dropdown menu, choose *non-parametric tests* from that, and click on *test for several independent samples*. The resulting dialogue box is as given below:

The variables repeat1, repeat2, and repeat3 are transferred to the right-hand side box named "test variable list." Now, click on OK to run the analysis. The output produced is as given below:

Ranks

	Mean Rank
REPEAT1	1.60
REPEAT2	1.80
REPEAT3	2.60

Test Statistics[a]

N	5
Chi-Square	2.800
df	2
Asymp. Sig.	.247

a. Friedman Test

22.4   RUNNING "CORRELATION ANALYSIS AND REGRESSION ANALYSIS"(METHODS IN CHAPTER 12)

22.4.1   RUNNING "PEARSON CORRELATION COEFFICIENT"

The marks scored in mathematics (mathes) and in statistics (stat) by a group of five students are as given in the following data editor.

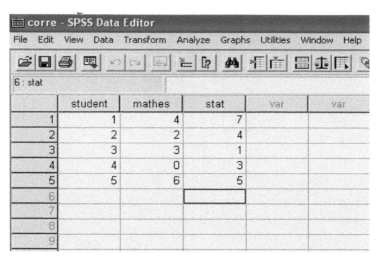

We wish to compute the Pearson correlation coefficient between the scores of mathematics and statistics using SPSS.

22.4.1.1   MAIN DIALOGUE BOX

Click on *analyze*, which will produce a dropdown menu, choose *correlate* from it, and then click on *bivariate correlation*. The resultant dialogue box is as shown below:

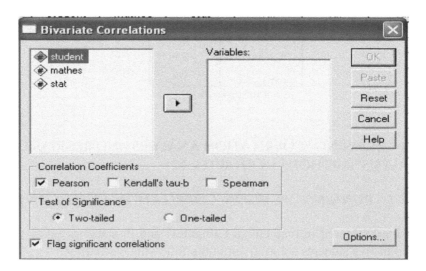

The default selection is Pearson correlation coefficient. Click on OK to run the analysis. The output produced is as shown below:

Correlations

		MATHES	STAT
MATHES	Pearson Correlation	1	.450
	Sig. (2-tailed)	.	.447
	N	5	5
STAT	Pearson Correlation	.450	1
	Sig. (2-tailed)	.447	.
	N	5	5

22.4.2 RUNNING "LINEAR REGRESSION ANALYSIS"

The "dosage" of a drug given to a group of five patients and their "improvement score" are as given in the following data editor.

🖿 Untitled - SPSS Data Editor

File Edit View Data Transform Analyze Graphs Utilities Window Help

6 : improve

	patient	dosage	improve	var	var	var
1	1	4	7			
2	2	2	4			
3	3	3	1			
4	4	0	3			
5	5	6	5			
6						
7						
8						

We wish to carry out linear regression analysis between the dependent variable (improvement) and the independent variable (dosage).

22.4.2.1 MAIN DIALOGUE BOX

Click on *analyze*, which will produce a drop down menu, choose *regression* from that, and click on *linear* as shown in the following dialogue box.

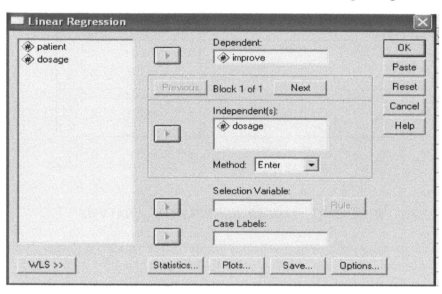

Transfer the dependent variable (improvement score) into the right-hand side box labeled "Dependent." Transfer the independent variable (dosage) into the box labeled "Independent(s)." We transfer the student into the box "Case Labels." In the main dialogue box, there are several buttons for advanced users. The "Save" button can be used to save statistics but predicted values and residuals.

Click on OK in the main dialogue box to run the analysis. The output produced has several tables. We are interested in the following output-tables.

Coefficients[a]

Model		Unstandardized Coefficients		Standardized Coefficients		
		B	Std. Error	Beta	t	Sig.
1	(Constant)	2.650	1.859		1.426	.249
	DOSAGE	.450	.516	.450	.873	.447

a. Dependent Variable: IMPROVE

22.5 RUNNING "RELIABILITY ANALYSIS AND VALIDITY ANALYSIS"(METHODS IN CHAPTER 13)

22.5.1 RUNNING "CRONBACH'S ALPHA"

The assessment scores of the services rendered by a mental institute by five raters on three items are as given in the following data editor:

	rater	item1	item2	item3	var	var
alphadata - SPSS Data Editor						
6 : item3						
1	1	4	7	10		
2	2	2	4	7		
3	3	3	1	8		
4	4	0	3	6		
5	5	6	5	4		
6						
7						
8						
9						
10						

We wish to calculate Cronbach's alpha to measure whether all the three items measure the same dimension.

22.5.1.1 MAIN DIALOGUE BOX

Click on *analyze,* which will produce drop down menu, choose *scale* from that, and click on *reliability analysis.* The resultant dialogue box is as shown below:

The items from 1 to 3 are transferred to the right-hand side box named "Items." Click on OK to run the analysis. The output produced is as shown below:

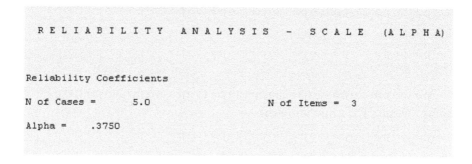

```
  R E L I A B I L I T Y    A N A L Y S I S   -   S C A L E    (A L P H A)


Reliability Coefficients

N of Cases =      5.0                  N of Items =  3

Alpha =    .3750
```

22.6   RUNNING "SURVIVAL ANALYSIS AND TIME SERIES ANALYSIS" (METHODS IN CHAPTER 14)

22.6.1   RUNNING "LIFE TABLES"

The duration of stay (DOS) of a group of 20 patients discharged in a psychiatric emergency ward are as given in the following data editor. We have only one value for status:1 representing discharge.

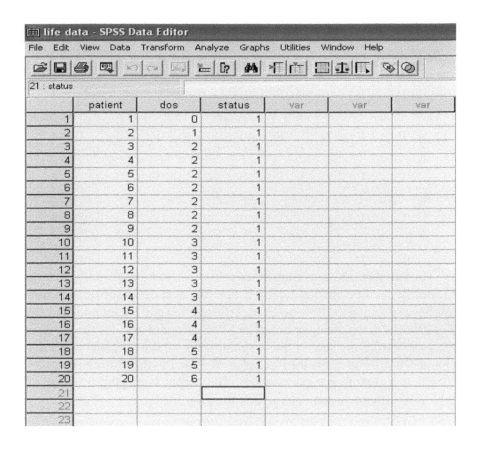

We wish to construct current hospital stay table for the data.

22.6.1.1   MAIN DIALOGUE BOX

Click on *analyze,* which will produce a drop down menu, choose *survival analysis* from that, and click on *life table*. The resultant dialogue box is as shown below:

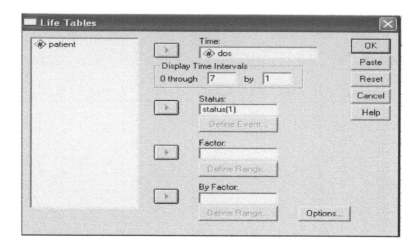

The variable (DOS) is transferred to the box named "Time." We have to specify the time interval for our data in the next down specified button. We have specified the time range as 7 (through 7) and the internal as 1 (by 1) as shown in the dialogue box. The SPSS program asks for the status of the patient after the stay in the hospital, since all the 20 patients are discharged and 1 represents the discharge. We put 1 in the status box.

Click on OK to run the analysis. The output is displayed in several tables. We are interested only in the following life table.

```
This subfile contains:      20 observations

 Life Table
   Survival Variable  DOS


          Number  Number  Number  Number                   Cumul
 Intrvl   Entrng  Wdrawn  Exposd    of    Propn   Propn    Propn   Proba-
 Start     this   During    to    Termnl  Termi-  Sur-     Surv    bility  Hazard
 Time     Intrvl  Intrvl   Risk   Events  nating  viving  at End  Densty   Rate
 ------   ------  ------  ------  ------   ------  ------  ------  ------  ------
    .0     20.0     .0    20.0     1.0    .0500   .9500   .9500   .0500   .0513
   1.0     19.0     .0    19.0     1.0    .0526   .9474   .9000   .0500   .0541
   2.0     18.0     .0    18.0     7.0    .3889   .6111   .5500   .3500   .4828
   3.0     11.0     .0    11.0     5.0    .4545   .5455   .3000   .2500   .5882
   4.0      6.0     .0     6.0     3.0    .5000   .5000   .1500   .1500   .6667
   5.0      3.0     .0     3.0     2.0    .6667   .3333   .0500   .1000  1.0000
   6.0      1.0     .0     1.0     1.0   1.0000   .0000   .0000   .0500  2.0000

 The median survival time for these data is    3.20
```

22.6.2 RUNNING "SEQUENCE CHART"

Let us assume that the monthly number of registrations of psychiatric disorders in a health clinic are as given in Chapter 14.2.2.5 is entered in the data editor. We wish to draw a sequence chart in order to configurate the time series components of the data.

22.6.2.1 MAIN DIALOGUE BOX

Click on *graph menu*, which will produce dropdown menu, select, and click *sequence*. The resultant dialogue box is as shown below:

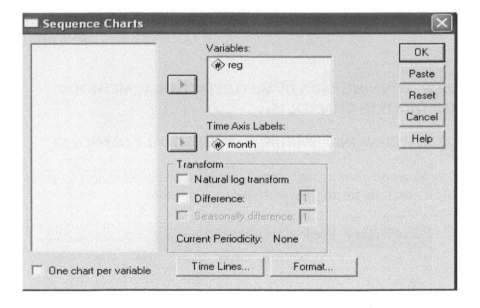

Click on OK to run the analysis. The output is displayed as follows:

22.7   RUNNING "MULTIVARIATE STATISTICAL METHODS" (METHODS IN CHAPTER 15)

22.7.1   RUNNING "PARTIAL CORRELATION COEFFICIENT"

The scores obtained in mathematics, statistics, and psychology of a group of five students are as given in the data editor below:

We wish to carry out partial correlation between mathes and statistics after eliminating the influence of psychology.

22.7.1.1 MAIN DIALOGUE BOX

Click on analyze, which will produce a drop down menu, choose correlation from that and click on 'partial…' resulting a dialogue box as shown below:

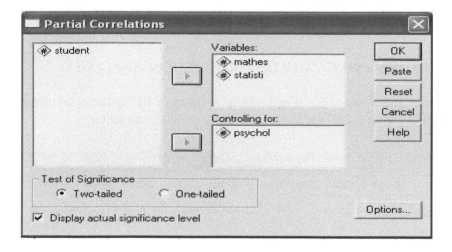

Transfer the variables mathes and statistics to the box labeled "Variables," and psychology to the box labeled "Controlling for" as shown in the dialogue box.

Click on OK in the main dialogue box to run the analysis. The output produced has several tables. We are interested in the following output table.

```
- - -  P A R T I A L    C O R R E L A T I O N    C O E F F I C I E N T S

Controlling for..    PSYCHOL

                MATHES    STATISTI

MATHES          1.0000      .4955
                (    0)    (    2)
                P= .       P= .504

STATISTI         .4955     1.0000
                (    2)    (    0)
                P= .504    P= .

(Coefficient / (D.F.) / 2-tailed Significance)

" . " is printed if a coefficient cannot be computed
```

22.7.2 RUNNING "MULTIPLE REGRESSION ANALYSIS"

The IQ and dosage of a drug given to a group of five patients and their "improvement score" are as given in the following data editor:

	patient	iq	dosage	improvem	var
1	1	91	4	7	
2	2	100	2	4	
3	3	109	3	1	
4	4	97	0	3	
5	5	103	6	5	
6					
7					

mradata - SPSS Data Editor

File Edit View Data Transform Analyze Graphs Utilities Window Help

6 : improvem

We wish to carry out multiple regression analysis between the dependent variable(improvement) and the Independent variables(IQ and dosage).

22.7.2.1 MAIN DIALOGUE BOX

Click on *analyze*, which will produce a dropdown menu, choose *regression* from that and click on *linear*... resulting a dialogue box as shown below.

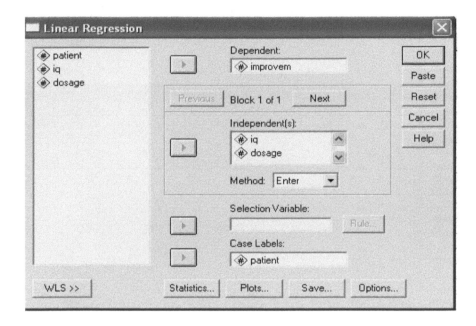

Transfer the dependent variable 'Improvement' into the right-hand side box labeled "Dependent." Transfer the independent variables (IQ and dosage) into the box labeled "Independent(s)." We transfer the patient into the box "Case Labels." In the main dialogue box, there are several buttons for advanced users. The save button can be used to save statistics such as predicted values and residuals.

Click on OK in the main dialogue box to run the analysis. The output produced has several tables. We are interested in the following output tables.

Coefficients[a]

Model		Unstandardized Coefficients		Standardized Coefficients	t	Sig.
		B	Std. Error	Beta		
1	(Constant)	31.833	3.932		8.097	.015
	IQ	-.296	.040	-.887	-7.466	.017
	DOSAGE	.583	.119	.583	4.906	.039

a. Dependent Variable: IMPROVEM

---

mradata - SPSS Data Editor

File   Edit   View   Data   Transform   Analyze   Graphs   Utilities   Window   Help

6 : improvem

	patient	iq	dosage	improvem	pre_1	res_1	var
1	1	91	4	7	7.246	-.246	
2	2	100	2	4	3.417	.583	
3	3	109	3	1	1.338	-.338	
4	4	97	0	3	3.138	-.138	
5	5	103	6	5	4.862	.138	
6							
7							

22.8   RUNNING "CLUSTER ANALYSIS AND DISCRIMINANT ANALYSIS" (METHODS IN CHAPTERS 16 AND 17)

22.8.1   RUNNING "HIERARCHICAL CLUSTER ANALYSIS"

The scores of 6 patients on two diagnostic tests are as given in the following data editor:

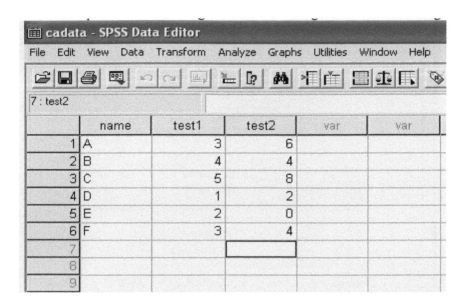

We wish to carry out cluster analysis in order to make groups of similar patients (diagnoses). We have planned to carry out hierarchical agglomerative cluster analysis using squared Euclidian distance employing nearest neighborhood method in order to get two clusters.

22.8.1.1   MAIN DIALOGUE BOX

Click on *analyze*, which will produce a dropdown menu, choose *classify* from that, and click on *hierarchical cluster*. The resultant dialogue box is as shown in the figure below:

The two numerical variables (test1, test2) are transferred to the right-hand side box named "Variable(s)." The patient name labeled "Name" is transferred to the box labeled "Label Cases by." There are four buttons for advanced users. We will use the statistics button to select proximity matrix, and cluster membership as a single solution with 2 clusters. We can use "Plot" button to select dendrogram. We can use "Method" button to select neighbor method. Finally, we can use the "Save" button to save the cluster membership in the data editor.

Click on OK to run the analysis. The SPSS display cluster analysis output in many tables. We are presenting only the following output tables.

Proximity Matrix

Case	Squared Euclidean Distance					
	1:A	2:B	3:C	4:D	5:E	6:F
1:A	.000	5.000	8.000	20.000	37.000	4.000
2:B	5.000	.000	17.000	13.000	20.000	1.000
3:C	8.000	17.000	.000	52.000	73.000	20.000
4:D	20.000	13.000	52.000	.000	5.000	8.000
5:E	37.000	20.000	73.000	5.000	.000	17.000
6:F	4.000	1.000	20.000	8.000	17.000	.000

This is a dissimilarity matrix

Cluster membership and dendrogram

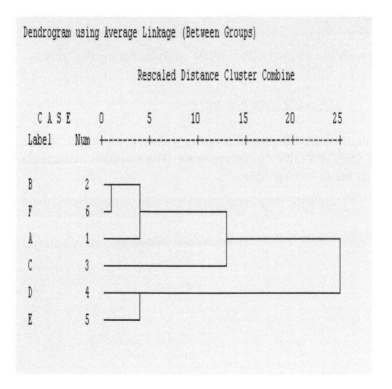

22.8.2   *RUNNING "LINEAR DISCRIMINANT ANALYSIS"*

The scores of two diagnostic groups of patients on two diagnostic criterion tests are as given in the following data editor:

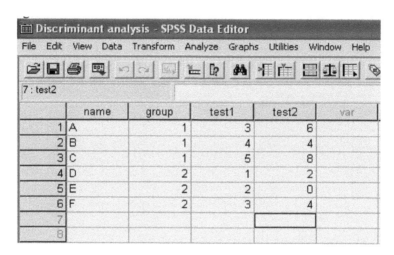

We wish to carry out discriminate analysis for the two groups.

22.8.2.1   *MAIN DIALOGUE BOX*

Click on *analyze*, which will produce a dropdown menu, choose *classify* from that, and click on *discriminate*. The resultant dialogue box is as shown in the following table:

The group variable is transferred to the right-hand side box named "Grouping Variable." The two-independent variables (test1, test2) are transferred to the right-hand side box named "Independents." There are buttons for advanced users. We use only the "Save" button and select(1) predicted group membership,(2) discriminant score, and (3) probabilities of group membership. SPSS display discriminant analysis output in many tables. But we are interested only in the predicted group membership, scores, and probability of group membership. These results are saved in the data editor window as shown below:

	name	group	test1	test2	dis_1	dis1_1	dis1_2	dis2_2
1	A	1	3	6	1	.57735	.79139	.20861
2	B	1	4	4	1	.57735	.79139	.20861
3	C	1	5	8	1	2.30940	.99520	.00480
4	D	2	1	2	2	-1.73205	.01799	.98201
5	E	2	2	0	2	-1.73205	.01799	.98201
6	F	2	3	4	1	.00000	.50000	.50000
7								
8								

22.9 RUNNING "FACTOR ANALYSIS" (METHODS IN CHAPTER 18)

22.9.1 RUNNING "PRINCIPAL COMPONENT ANALYSIS"

The marks scored in mathematics (mathes), statistics (stat), and in psychology (psycho) by a group of five students are as given in the following data editor:

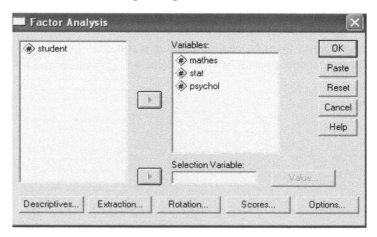

We wish to carry out factor analysis in order to reduce the 3 variables data into 2-dimensional (factors) without losing much information. We are planning to use correlation matrix and apply principal components analysis method of extraction of factors, and by applying varimax method of factor rotations.

22.9.1.1   MAIN DIALOGUE BOX

Click on *analyze,* which will produce a dropdown menu, choose data *reduction* from that, and click on *factor analysis.* The resultant dialogue box is as shown in the following dialogue box.

The three variables are transferred to the box named variables. In this main dialogue box, there are five buttons for advance users. We will use the descriptive button to display the correlation coefficient matrix. The extraction button is used to specify the number of factors (3 in our example). The default settings are for principal components. Finally, the "Rotation" button is used to specify method of rotation (varimax). Click on OK to run the analysis. The SPSS display factor analysis output in many tables. Only the following table is presented.

Factor Analysis

Correlation Matrix

		MATHES	STATISTI	PSYCHOLO
Correlation	MATHES	1.000	.765	-.482
	STATISTI	.765	1.000	-.271
	PSYCHOLO	-.482	-.271	1.000

Rotated Component Matrix[a]

	Component		
	1	2	3
MATHES	.463	-.274	.843
STATISTI	.925	-.105	.364
PSYCHOLO	-.104	.975	-.197

Extraction Method: Principal Component Analysis.

KEYWORDS

- **Cronbach's Alpha**
- **Duration of stay**
- **One-way ANOVA**
- **t-test**

BIBLIOGRAPHY

STATISTICAL METHODS (CHAPTERS 1–20)

1. Sundar Rao, P. S. S.; and Richard, J.; An Introduction to Biostatistics: A Manual For students in Health Sciences (third edition). New Delhi: Prentice-Hall of India; **1999**.
2. Bailley, N. T. J.; Statistical Methods in Biology. New York: Cambridge University Press; **1994**.
3. Reddy, M. V.; Statistics for Mental Health Care Research. Bangalore: NIMHANS Publications; **2002**.
4. Dunn, G.; Statistics in Psychiatry. London: Arnold; **2000**.
5. Banerjee, S; and Roy, R.; Fundamentals of Research Methodology. Allahabad: Kitab Mahal; **2008**.
6. Rajagopal, V.; Selected Statistical Tests. New Delhi: New Age International; **2006**.
7. Dawson, B; and Trapp, R. G.; Basic and Clinical Biostatistics. New York: McGraw Hill (Fourth Edition); **2004**.
8. Siegel, S.; Non-Parametric Statistics for the Behavioral Sciences. New York: Mc-Graw-Hill: **1988**.
9. Hope, K.; Methods of Multivariate Analysis. London: University of London Press; **1968**.
10. Everitt, B. S.; Medical Statistics from A to Z. New York: Cambridge University Press; **2009**.
11. Reddy, M. V.; and Chandrasekhar, C. R.; Prevalence of mental and behavioral disorders in India: a meta-analysis. *Indian J. Psyc.* **1998**, *40*, 149–157.
12. Bartko, J. J.; and Carpenter, W. T.; On the methods and theory of reliability. *J. Nerv. Ment Dis.* **1976**, *163*, 307–317.
13. Hanji, M. B.; Meta-Analytical Approach to Estimate Pattern of Prevalence of Schizophrenia and Epilepsy in India PhD Dissertation. Bangalore: National Institute of Mental Health and Neurosciences (NIMHANS); **2007**.
14. Suresh, K. P.; Evaluation of clustering methods for pattern recognisation in scholastic improvement of rural children, Ph.D. Dissertation. Bangalore: National Institute of Mental Health and Neurosciences (NIMHANS); **2008**.

STATISTICAL PACKAGE FOR SOCIAL SCIENCES SPSS (CHAPTERS 21 AND 22)

15. Gour, A. S.; and Gour, S. S.; Statistical Methods for Practice and Research. New Delhi: Response Books (Sage Publications); **2006**.

16. Kerr, A. W.; Hall, H. K.; and Kozub,S. A.; Doing Statistics with SPSS. New Delhi: Sage Publications; **2002**.

17. Field, A.; Discovering Statistics Using SPSS. New York: Sage Publications; **2007**.

18. Carver, R. H; and Nash, J. G.; Doing data Analysis with SPSS Version 14. Belmont: Thomson Brook Cole; **2006**.

APPENDIX

APPENDIX I: BASIC DATA OF 40 REGISTERED PATIENTS AT NIMHANS

Registration number	Serial number	Age	Sex	Marital status	Locality	Diagnosis (ICD-10)
293307	1	60	Male	Married	Rural	32.3
293308	2	80	Female	Single	Rural	00.1
293309	3	4	Female	Single	Urban	80.0
293310	4	22	Female	Single	Rural	34.0
293311	5	26	Male	Married	Rural	23.0
293312	6	21	Male	Single	Rural	20.3
293313	7	23	Female	Married	Rural	32.3
293314	8	25	Male	Single	Rural	20.3
293315	9	29	Male	Married	Urban	42.0
293316	10	9	Female	Single	Urban	81.3
293317	11	51	Male	Married	Rural	44.5
293318	12	31	Female	Married	Semi-urban	34.1
293319	13	48	Female	Married	Rural	41.1
293320	14	25	Female	Single	Rural	32.3
293321	15	65	Male	Married	Semi-urban	29.0
293322	16	12	Male	Single	Rural	81.3
293323	17	16	Female	Single	Rural	70.0
293324	18	13	Male	Single	Urban	70.0
293325	19	29	Male	Married	Urban	31.1

Registration number	Serial number	Age	Sex	Marital status	Locality	Diagnosis (ICD-10)
293326	20	76	Male	Married	rural	31.4
293327	21	12	Male	Single	Semi-urban	90.0
293328	22	10	Male	Single	Rural	81.3
293329	23	35	Male	Married	Semi-urban	10.3
293330	24	40	Male	Married	Semi-urban	20.0
293331	25	11	Male	Single	Urban	44.9
293332	26	70	Male	Married	Urban	31.0
293333	27	24	Female	Single	Urban	43.0
293334	28	58	Female	Married	Semi-urban	00.0
293335	29	60	Female	Married	Semi-urban	23.0
293336	30	27	Male	Single	Semi-urban	30.1
293337	31	30	Male	Single	Semi-urban	43.2
293338	32	50	Female	Single	Rural	29.0
293339	33	26	Male	Single	Semi-urban	31.0
293340	34	25	Male	Single	Semi-urban	29.0
293341	35	27	Male	Single	Urban	42.0
293342	36	19	Male	Single	Urban	31.8
293343	37	33	Female	Married	Urban	33.0
293344	38	35	Male	Single	Rural	34.1
293345	39	24	Female	Married	Semi-urban	31.6
293346	40	44	Female	Married	Semi-urban	33.1

APPENDIX II—CLASSIFICATION OF STATISTICAL METHODS

CHAPTER 1: PSYCHIATRIC RESEARCH

1.1 RESEARCH QUESTIONS IN PSYCHIATRY
Recognition
Diagnosis
Treatment
Prevention

1.2 RESEARCH APPROACHES
(1) Scientific Approach
Features
Steps
Science and psychiatry
(2) Mill's Canons
Method of difference
Method of agreement
Joint method of difference and agreement
Method of concomitant variation
Method of residues
(3) Qualitative Research
(4) Quantitative Research

1.3 PROTOCOL WRITING FOR QUANTITATIVE STUDIES
(1) The Research Question
Review of literature
Need for the study
Aims and objectives
(2) Type of Study
(3) Plan of Study
Population
Variables
Standardization
Experimental settings (if any)
Record form
Response error
Non-response error
(4) Plan of Analysis
Statistical methods
Database and data analysis software
(5) Reporting the Results

1.4 VARIABLES IN PSYCHIATRY
(1) Nature of Variables in Psychiatry

(2) Qualitative Variables and Quantitative Variables
(3) Levels of Measurement of Variables
     Nominal level
     Ordinal level
     Interval level
     Ratio level
(4) Further Types of Variables
     Independent and dependent variables
     Covariates
     Concomitant variables
     Factors/dimensions
(5) Discrete and Continuous Data

1.5 STATISTICAL METHODS IN PSYCHIATRIC RESEARCH
(1) Organization and Collection of Data
     Observational studies (Chapter 2)
     Experimental studies (Chapter 3)
(2) Descriptive Statistics
     One-variable descriptive statistics (Chapter 4)
     Mental health statistics (Chapter 5)
(3) Basis of Statistical Inference
     Probability and probability distributions (Chapter 6)
     Sampling theory and methods (Chapter 7)
     Basic elements of statistical Inference (Chapter 8)
(4) Tests of Significance of Hypotheses
     Parametric tests of significance (Chapter 9)
     Experimental data analysis: ANOVA (Chapter 10)
     Non-parametric tests of significance (Chapter 11)
(5) Correlational Variables Data Analysis
     Correlational analysis and regression analysis (Chapter 12)
     Reliability analysis and validity analysis (Chapter 13)
     Survival analysis and time series analysis (Chapter 14)
(6) Multivariate Data Analysis
     Multivariate statistical methods (Chapter 15)
     Cluster analysis (Chapter 16)
     Discriminant analysis (Chapter 17)
     Factor analysis (Chapter 18)
(7) Multi-study Data-Points Analysis Meta-analysis (Chapter 19)

CHAPTER 2: OBSERVATIONAL STUDIES

2.1 CASE-SERIES ANALYSIS
Observational units
Variables
Record form

2.2 CROSS-SECTIONAL STUDIES
(1) Hospital In-Patients Census
     Observational units
     Variables
     Record form
(2) Mental Morbidity Studies
     Observational units
     Variables
     Household information schedule
     Socio-economic status schedule
     Case detection schedule
     Case record schedule

2.3 LONGITUDINAL STUDIES
(1) Retrospective Studies
     Schematic representation
     Patient group and normal control group
     Suspected risk/causal factors
     Record form
(2) Prospective Studies
     Schematic representation
     With risk subjects and without risk subjects
     Anticipated disease
     Record form

CHAPTER 3: EXPERIMENTAL STUDIES

3.1 BASIC ELEMENTS OF EXPERIMENTS
(1) Experimental Error
(2) Basic Principles of Experiments
     Replication
     Randomization
     Local control
(3) Laboratory Experiments and Clinical Experiments
(4) Therapeutic Trials and Prophylactic Trials
(5) Uncontrolled and Controlled Trials

4.2 GRAPHICAL REPRESENTATION OF CLASSIFIED DATA
- (1) Qualitative Variable Data
  Bar diagram
- (2) Quantitative Variable Data
  Frequency polygon
  Histogram

4.3 Summarizing Data: Averages
- (1) Quantitative Variable Data
  Mean
  Median
  Mode
- (2) Qualitative Variable Data
  Proportion and percentage
  Rate and ratio
  Indicators and index

4.4 SUMMARIZING DATA: DISPERSION
- (1) Quantitative Variable Data
  Range
  Standard deviation
  Coefficient of variation
- (2) Qualitative Variable Data
  Frequency distribution

4.5 SUMMARIZING DATA: SKEWNESS AND KURTOSIS
- (1) Skewness
  Coefficient of skewness
- (2) Kurtosis

4.6 DESCRIPTIVE STATISTICS FOR SPATIAL DATA
Classification of spatial data
Spot maps
Density of patients

4.7 Descriptive Statistics for Time-Related Data
Classification of time-related data
Epidemiological curves
Expectation of duration of time and Time series components

CHAPTER 5: MENTAL HEALTH STATISTICS

5.1 DEMOGRAPHIC INDICATORS
- (1) Population Size
  Malthus theory
- (2) Population Composition

(3) Normal Distribution
     Central limit theorem
(4) Standard Errors of Statistics
     Standard error of sample mean
     Standard error of sample proportion
(5) Derived Distributions
     Standardized values
     χ^2 (Chi-squared) distribution
     t-Distribution
     F-Distribution

CHAPTER 7: SAMPLING THEORY AND METHODS

7.1 Theory of Sampling
Random sampling
Non-random sampling
Sampling error
Sampling bias
7.2 RANDOM SAMPLING METHODS
(1) Simple Random Sampling
     Estimate
     Random numbers
(2) Systematic Sampling
     Estimate
(3) Stratified Sampling
     Estimate
(4) Cluster Sampling
     Estimate
(5) Area Sampling
7.3 RANDOM SAMPLING METHODS IN MENTAL MORBIDITY SURVEYS
Rural sectors
Urban sectors
Semi-urban sectors

CHAPTER 8: BASIC ELEMENTS OF STATISTICAL INFERENCE

8.1 BASIC ELEMENTS OF ESTIMATION OF PARAMETERS
(1) Point Estimates
     Consistency, efficiency, and sufficiency

CHAPTER 10: EXPERIMENTAL DATA ANALYSIS: ANOVA

10.1 One-Way ANOVA
Layout
Hypotheses
Technique
Test statistic
ANOVA table
10.2 Post-Hoc Multiple Comparison Tests: *Scheffé's method*
Hypotheses
Critical value of F
Test statistics
10.3 Two-Way ANOVA
Layout
Hypotheses
Technique
Test statistic
ANOVA table
10.4 Factorial ANOVA
Layout
Hypotheses
Technique
Test statistic
2^2-Factorial ANOVA table
10.5 Repeated Measures ANOVA
Layout
Hypotheses
Technique
Test statistic
Repeated measures ANOVA table

CHAPTER 11: NON-PARAMETRIC TESTS OF SIGNIFICANCE

11.1 ONE-SAMPLE NON-PARAMETRIC TESTS
(1)   Chi-square Tests: $1 \times k$ Contingency Table
        Hypotheses
        $1 \times k$ contingency table
        Test statistic
(2)   Chi-square Tests: $r \times k$ Contingency Table
        Hypotheses
        $r \times k$ contingency table

Test statistic
(3) Chi-square Tests: 2 × 2 Contingency Table
     Hypotheses
     2 × 2 contingency table
     Test statistic
(4) Chi-square Tests: 2 × k Contingency table
     Hypotheses
     2 × k contingency table
     Test statistic
(5) Tests of Significance of Individual Cell Frequencies
     Hypotheses
     Contingency table
     Test statistics
(6) One-Sample Run-Test
     Hypotheses
     Sequence of events
     Test statistic

11.2 TWO INDEPENDENT SAMPLE NON-PARAMETRIC TESTS
(1) Median Test
(2) Mann–Whitney U-test
     Hypotheses
     Mann–Whitney U-test table
     Test statistic

11.3 TWO RELATED SAMPLE NON-PARAMETRIC TESTS
(1) McNemar's Test
     Hypotheses
     McNemar's test table
     Test statistic
(2) Sign Test
     Hypotheses
     Sign test table
     Test statistic

11.4 K-INDEPENDENT SAMPLE NON-PARAMETRIC TESTS
(1) Extended Median Test
(2) Krushkal–Wallis H-test
     Hypotheses
     Krushkal–Wallis H-test table
     Test statistic

11.5 K-RELATED SAMPLE NON-PARAMETRIC TESTS
(1) Cochran Q-test
     Hypotheses
     Cochran Q-test table

CHAPTER 19: META-ANALYSIS

19.1 LOCATION AND SELECTION OF STUDIES FOR META-ANALYSIS
(1) Location of Studies
     Publication bias
(2) Selection of Studies
19.2 END-POINTS OF PRIMARY STUDIES
(1) A List of End-Points
     Cohen's *d*
(2) Transformation of End-Points
19.3 QUALITY ASSESSMENT OF SELECTED STUDIES
(1) A List of Quality Assessment Items
(2) Internal Validity and External Validity
19.4 META-ANALYSIS MASTER SHEET
Statistical heterogeneity and clinical heterogeneity
19.5 Meta-Analysis Plots
Forest plot
Funnel plot
19.6 METHODS FOR POOLING END-POINTS: FIXED EFFECTS MODEL
(1) Fixed Effects Model
(2) Sample-Size Method
     Pooled estimate
(3) Inverse-Variance Method
     Pooled estimate
(4) Heterogeneity Statistics
19.7 METHODS FOR POOLING END-POINTS: RANDOM EFFECTS MODEL
(1) Random Effects Model
(2) DL Method
     Pooled estimate
19.8 ADDITIONAL META-ANALYSIS TECHNIQUES
Sensitivity meta-analysis technique
Influence meta-analysis technique
Sub-group meta-analysis technique
Cumulative meta-analysis technique
19.9 IMPLICATIONS OF THE RESULTS OF META-ANALYSIS
Research implications
Clinical implications
Economic implications

Implications for policy making
Numerical demonstration

CHAPTER 20: REPORTING THE RESULTS

20.1 EVALUATION OF THE STUDY
    (1) Data Description
    (2) Internal Validity and External Validity
    (3) Comparison with Other Evidences
20.2 INTERPRETING THE RESULTS
    (1) Dataset
    (2) Descriptive Statistics
    (3) Statistical Inference
20.3 WRITING THE REPORT
    (1) Major Criticisms
    (2) Writing Scientific Papers
    (3) Writing Technical Reports
    (4) Reporting Data Analysis
    (5) Reporting the Results

CHAPTER 21: STATISTICAL PACKAGE FOR SOCIAL SCIENCES

21.1 SPSS DATA EDITOR
    (1) Menu Items
          File, edit, and view
          Data and transform
          Analyze and graph
          Utility, window, and help
    (2) Further Items
21.2 PROCEDURES FOR ENTERING DATA IN SPSS
    (1) Name
    (2) Type, Width, and Decimal
    (3) Value and Label
    (4) Further Items
    (5) Saving the File
21.3 PROCEDURES FOR RUNNING DATA ANALYSIS USING SPSS
    (1) Dataset and Data Editor Format
    (2) Plan of Analysis
    (3) Main Dialogue Box
    (4) Output

21.4 DATA HANDLING USING DATA MENU
   (1)   Split File
         Main dialogue box
   (2)   Weight Cases
         Main dialogue box
21.5 DATA HANDLING USING TRANSFORM MENU
   (1)   Recode
         Main dialogue box

CHAPTER 22: RUNNING DATA ANALYSIS USING SPSS

22.1 RUNNING "PARAMETRIC TESTS OF SIGNIFICANCE" (METHODS IN CHAPTER 9)
   (1)   Running "One-Sample t-Test"
         Main dialogue box
   (2)   Running "Independent Samples t-Test"
         Main dialogue box
   (3)   Running "Paired-Sample t-test"
         Main dialogue box
22.2 RUNNING "ANOVA TESTS" (METHODS IN CHAPTER 10)
   (1)   Running "One-Way ANOVA"
         Main dialogue box
   (2)   Running "ANCOVA Test"
         Main dialogue box
   (3)   Running "Repeated Measures ANOVA"
         Main dialogue box
22.3 RUNNING "NON-PARAMETRIC TESTS OF SIGNIFICANCE" (METHODS IN CHAPTER 11)
   (1)   Running "Chi-Square Test of Significance"
         Main dialogue box
   (2)   Running "Run Test"
         Main dialogue box
   (3)   Running "Mann–Whitney U-Test"
         Main dialogue box
   (4)   Running "Krushkal–Wallis H-Test"
         Main dialogue box
   (5)   Running "Friedman Test"
         Main dialogue box
22.4 RUNNING "CORRELATION ANALYSIS AND REGRESSION ANALYSIS" "(METHODS IN CHAPTER 12)
   (1)   Running "Pearson Correlation Coefficient'

Main dialogue box
(2) Running "Linear Regression Analysis"
Main dialogue box

22.5 RUNNING "RELIABILITY ANALYSIS" (METHODS IN CHAPTER 13)
(1) Running "Cronbach's Alpha"
Main dialogue box

22.6 RUNNING "SURVIVAL ANALYSIS AND TIME SERIES ANALYSIS" (METHODS IN CHAPTER 14)
(1) Running "Life Tables"
Main dialogue box
(2) Running "Sequence Chart"
Main dialogue box

22.7 RUNNING "MULTIVARIATE STATISTICAL METHODS" (METHODS IN CHAPTER 15)
(1) Running "Partial Correlation Coefficient"
Main dialogue box
(2) Running "Multiple Regression Analysis"
Main dialogue box

22.8 RUNNING "CLUSTER ANALYSIS AND DISCRIMINANT ANALYSIS" (METHODS IN CHAPTERS 16 AND 17)
(1) Running "Hierarchical Cluster Analysis"
Main dialogue box
(2) Running "Linear Discriminant Analysis"
Main dialogue box

22.9 RUNNING "FACTOR ANALYSIS" (METHODS IN CHAPTER 18)
(1) Running "Principal Component Analysis"
Main dialogue box

APPENDIX III: PROBABILITY DISTRIBUTION TABLES

Area under the standard normal curve (Z-values)

Normal deviate (Z)	.00	.02	.04	.06	.08
0.0	.000	.008	.016	.024	.032
0.1	.040	.048	.056	.064	.071
0.2	.079	.087	.095	.103	.110
0.3	.118	.126	.133	.141	.148
0.4	.155	.163	.170	.177	.184
0.5	.192	.199	.205	.212	.219
0.6	.226	.232	.239	.245	.252
0.7	.258	.264	.270	.276	.282
0.8	.288	.294	.299	.305	.311
0.9	.316	.321	.326	.332	.337
1.0	.341	.346	.351	.355	.360
1.1	.364	.369	.373	.377	.381
1.2	.385	.389	.393	.396	.400
1.3	.403	.407	.410	.413	.416
1.4	.419	.422	.425	.428	.431
1.5	.433	.436	.438	.441	.443
1.6	.445	.447	.450	.452	.454
1.7	.455	.457	.459	.461	.463
1.8	.464	.466	.467	.469	.470
1.9	.471	.473	.474	.475	.476
2.0	.477	.478	.479	.480	.481
2.1	.482	.483	.484	.485	.486
2.2	.486	.487	.488	.488	.489
2.3	.489	.490	.490	.491	.491
2.4	.492	.492	.493	.493	.493
2.5	.494	.494	.495	.495	.495
2.6	.495	.496	.496	.496	.496
2.7	.496	.497	.497	.497	.497
2.8	.497	.498	.498	.498	.498
2.9	.498	.498	.498	.499	.499
3.0	.499	.499	.499	.499	.499

Critical values of χ^2

Degrees of freedom (df)	Significance level (0.05)	Significance (0.01)
1	3.84	6.64
2	5.99	9.21
3	7.81	11.35
4	9.49	13.28
5	11.07	15.09
6	12.59	16.81
7	14.07	18.48
8	15.51	20.09
9	16.92	21.67
10	18.31	23.21
11	19.68	24.73
12	21.03	26.22
13	22.36	27.69
14	23.68	29.14
15	25.00	30.58
16	26.30	32.00
17	27.59	33.41
18	28.87	34.81
19	30.14	36.19
20	31.41	37.57
21	32.67	38.93
22	33.92	40.29
23	35.17	41.64
24	36.42	42.98
25	37.65	44.31
26	38.89	45.64
27	40.11	46.96
28	41.34	48.28
29	42.56	49.59
30	43.77	50.89

Critical values of t for two-tailed tests

Degrees of freedom (df)	Significance level (0.05)	Significance (0.01)
1	12.71	63.66
2	4.30	9.93
3	3.18	5.84
4	2.78	4.60
5	2.57	4.03
6	2.45	3.71
7	2.37	3.50
8	2.31	3.36
9	2.26	3.25
10	2.23	3.17
11	2.20	3.11
12	2.18	3.06
13	2.16	3.01
14	2.15	2.98
15	2.13	2.95
16	2.12	2.92
17	2.11	2.90
18	2.10	2.88
19	2.09	2.86
20	2.09	2.85
21	2.08	2.83
22	2.07	2.82
23	2.07	2.81
24	2.06	2.80
25	2.06	2.79
26	2.06	2.78
27	2.05	2.77
28	2.05	2.76
29	2.05	2.75
30	2.04	2.74

Critical values of F at 5% level of significance

df_1 df_2	1	2	3	4	5	6	7	8
1	161.00	200.00	216.00	225.00	230.00	234.00	237.00	239.00
2	18.51	19.00	19.16	19.25	19.30	19.33	19.35	19.37
3	10.13	9.55	9.28	9.12	9.01	8.94	8.89	8.85
4	7.71	6.94	6.59	6.39	6.26	6.16	6.09	6.04
6	5.99	5.14	4.76	4.53	4.39	4.28	4.21	4.15
8	5.32	4.46	4.07	3.84	3.69	3.58	3.50	3.44
10	4.96	4.10	3.71	3.48	3.33	3.22	3.14	3.07
12	4.75	3.89	3.49	3.26	3.11	3.00	2.91	2.85
14	4.60	3.74	3.34	3.11	2.96	2.85	2.76	2.70
16	4.49	3.63	3.24	3.01	2.85	2.74	2.66	2.59
18	4.41	3.55	3.16	2.93	2.77	2.66	2.58	2.51
20	4.35	3.49	3.10	2.87	2.71	2.60	2.51	2.45
30	4.17	3.32	2.92	2.69	2.53	2.42	2.33	2.27
40	4.08	3.23	2.84	2.61	2.45	2.34	2.25	2.18
50	4.03	3.18	2.79	2.56	2.40	2.29	2.20	2.13
60	4.00	3.15	2.76	2.53	2.37	2.25	2.17	2.10

INDEX